Keto Fl...

The 4 Secrets to Reduce Inflammation, Burn Fat & Reboot Your Metabolism

By

Ben Azadi

The information presented herein represents the views of the author as of the date of publication. This book is presented for informational purposes only. Due to the rate at which conditions change, the author reserves the right to alter and update his opinions at any time. While every attempt has been made to verify the information in this book, the author does not assume any responsibility for errors, inaccuracies, or omissions.

This book is not intended as a substitute for the medical advice of physicians. The reader should regularly consult a physician in matters relating to his/her health and particularly with respect to any symptoms that may require diagnosis or medical attention.

Praise for Keto Flex

"Ben Azadi has been a great resource to the low carb and fasting community. Ben's new book Keto Flex explores different applications of ways to diet and fasting because there's not a one size fits all approach when it comes to your health. Keto Flex provides the latest in research and practical strategies. This is a great read for understanding weight loss, health and longevity. "

- Dr Jason Fung
Best Selling Author of The Obesity Code

"We all want to be healthy and lean. And while there is no single variable that dictates metabolic health, the best evidence shows that the food we eat matters most. This is where Ben Azadi comes in. In the Keto Flex Diet, Ben lays out a strategy for drastically improving metabolic health with simple steps that involves adjusting not only what you eat, but also when you eat. If you're searching for a clearer view of your health, this book will provide the insight and strategy you've been looking for."

- Dr Benjamin Bikman
Author of Why We Get Sick

"Ben is one of the most trusted sources in the ketogenic community and Keto Flex simply makes sense. Our bodies have the ability to know how to regulate body fat, if we can just allow the ketogenic diet to do its part while letting the body do its part, we can live a flexible, non-restrictive lifestyle that gets our bodies and our emotions what they want! Go Ben! What a great Book!"

- Thomas A. DeLauer
Author, Health Expert & Performance Coach

"Ben Azadi is not only one of the smartest guys in the industry, but he's also a genius at breaking things down for people so that literally everyone can understand the step-by-step protocols he's put together to help others achieve optimal health. His book, Keto Flex, does just that! A super simple 4 step process that can't go wrong!"

- Drew Manning
NYT Best Selling Author

"In easy-to-follow, simple steps and rules, Ben Azadi provides you with a clear blueprint for everyone to take control of their waistline, blood sugar and other metabolic markers. These time-tested methods are simple, practical ways to regain control of your health using natural dietary methods instead of medications. "

- Megan Ramos
Clinical Researcher, author of Life in the Fasting Lane

"Ben Azadi is, without a doubt, one of the emerging leaders in the keto, low carb space.
His knowledge, enthusiasm and positivity are infectious and his take on ketogenic diets is refreshing. I love that Ben's approach takes into account bio-individuality and fully embraces finding your own path to wellness."

- Cynthia Thurlow
Nurse Practitioner, Women's Health Expert

"Ben is the most passionate and experienced keto gurus! His new book Keto Flex is a fantastic read for anyone interested in the keto diet! From the beginner to the experienced keto dieter, this book has the tips that will help you succeed!"

- Maria Emmerich
Best Selling Keto Author

"Ben Azadi is a daring soldier in the decades-long war against dietary lies that turn well-meaning doctors into unwitting agents of disease. Ben's track record of pulling casualties from the field and bringing them back to health should earn him some kind of nutritional purple heart. We need more strong voices like Ben's, and we need more books like Ben's Keto Flex."

- Cate Shanahan, MD
Author of NY Times Bestseller the FATBURN Fix

"Ben has come out with a great book about doing a sustainable ketogenic diet. Too often do authors and dieticians fall into the trap of their own dogma but Keto Flex circumvents that. Ben hits the nail on the head by implementing the concept of metabolic flexibility that allows the person to achieve optimal fat burning and glucose tolerance. I think every person should go through some periods of keto adaptation to prime their body for burning fat and ketones. However, it isn't necessary to stay in ketosis for the rest of your life to maintain those benefits. The steps outlined by Ben will help the person reach that state with ease and less stress. Besides the book, Ben is also working hard in inspiring people and helping them to transform their health."

- Siim Land
Author of Metabolic Autophagy

"Focusing on the balance of Fasting and Feasting is a powerful and ancestrally-informed strategy for transformation, vibrant health, and longevity. Since there is no magic bullet or one-size-fits-all approach, flexibility is critical to get results that last. We need Ben's insight and voice more than ever!"

- Abel James

New York Times Bestselling Author & Creator of Fat-Burning Man

"Ben has a unique way of taking a scientific approach yet breaking it down into easy, understandable, and most importantly, practical steps for you to apply on your keto journey. Keto Flex provides the latest science and applications for the ketogenic lifestyle with practical tips on how you can get started today. This is a must read for anyone looking to optimize their body and brain through ketogenic nutrition with practical advice on how to get started and sustain this lifestyle for years to come!"

- Ryan Lowery
Author of The Ketogenic Bible

"I am so thrilled Ben wrote this book! No one is more tenacious and thoughtful at empowering people to step into their greatness. In the ketogenic world, there has been a massive hole in information providing people the tools to properly move in and out of ketosis. Not only does Ben fill that hole with this book, but he eloquently lays out foundational principles of ketogenic diet that so many are missing. This book is a game changer for anyone wanting to build a ketogenic lifestyle!"

- Dr Mindy Pelz
Best Selling Author of The Menopause Reset

"Ben Azadi is one of the top thought leaders in the space of keto and intermittent fasting. His new book, Keto Flex, brings together the benefits of a low carb lifestyle, intermittent fasting, nutrient timing and carb cycling for optimal energy, fat burning and hormone balance. I highly recommend this book to anyone who wants to improve their brain and body!

- Dr David Jockers, DNM, DC, MS
Author of Keto Metabolic Breakthrough and The Fasting Transformation

Sustainability in your chosen diet requires three things: flexibility, creativity, and do-ability. Ben Azadi accomplishes all three of these brilliantly in his book, Keto Flex Lifestyle. Through countless hours of personal research, rigorous testing, and rugged innovation, he cuts to the heart of what it takes to get into and reap the benefits of a healthy state of nutritional ketosis—get adapted, introduce fasting, adjust to burning ketones, and flex in targeted and timed carbohydrates. With Keto Flex Lifestyle, Ben has crafted a usable plan of action that takes the concepts I shared about in my book Keto Clarity to the next level!

- Jimmy Moore
International bestselling author of Keto Clarity

Dedication

I want to dedicate this book to two amazing women in my life:
my mother Haddi Azadi and my girlfriend Natassia Coelho.

Mom, thank you for the tremendous support you to continue to
provide. You're the most unselfish person I've ever met in my life.
I love you.

Natassia, your support and love for me is daily oxygen for my
soul. I love you.

Contents

Foreword

This book is a true answer to the growing number of people who can't lose weight, have hit a weight plateau, have low energy or brain fog, or just want to take their health to the next level.

Many years ago, my wife and I both started a keto diet. Within days my ketones were soaring, and I felt amazing. The first thing I noticed was my brain clicked on, and I could recall facts and figures like never before. I felt like Superman, with boundless energy, and I even gained muscle and lost fat.

In contrast, my wife, Merily, did not experience the same success. Her ketones were barely getting over .4 to .5 (.8 to 1.8 is a good average for being in keto), and she was anything but thriving. I advised her to lower her carbs even more. That didn't work. Her energy declined and her ketones didn't move. I suggested that it might take her more time to adapt.

After a few months, it became clear this was not the case. Out of frustration and having no answers, I advised Merily to go back to a higher carb, healthy diet. She did, and felt better right away. After a month or two, I suggested she give it another try, and this time her ketones were a little better, and so too was her energy. That's when I came up with the idea to move her out of ketosis again for another month, and move her back in once again. The third time, it worked. She was thriving and her ketones were over 1.0 consistently.

After this experience, I decided to try this with some patients who were struggling in keto or just with weight loss resistance in general. It worked! Then I took the idea to my practitioners and doctors I coached, and asked them to try this "diet variation" concept, and the results were the same. Diet Variation was born. There are monthly and weekly strategies that work amazingly well for hormone challenged individuals such as thyroid, adrenal, and low hormones. The variation forces the body to adapt to the change, and it adapts by optimizing hormones.

Being one of my students, Ben took this concept, and he made it easy and usable for people to put into practice, as Ben does with most things. Keto Flex was born. This book is a user-friendly guide to a new concept in the low carb awakening that is sweeping the planet.

As it turns out, the concept is based on solid science. When you change your diet, even adding weekly feast days and famine days, the body must adapt to the abrupt changes, which leads to a "hormone optimization." Hormones are at the heart of why people stop losing weight, can't lose weight, or don't have success on a healthy diet when others do.

Recently I had the pleasure of interviewing Krista Varady, Ph.D., a professor of nutrition at the University of Illinois, Chicago. She discussed her studies on what she called "alternate day dieting." Her study compared many different diets with the concept of eating the standard American diet one day and then a diet of very restricted calories the next (feast/famine). The feast/famine worked better than all the other diets for weight loss. I asked why she thought this was the case, and she said, "It's all about adaptation." How does the body adapt? It optimizes our hormones, and the benefit is that we become more efficient fat burners. It's all about using the body's natural survival mechanisms. The #1 priority of the body is always survival. I have studied very healthy ancient cultures and have found that they were invariably forced into diet changes, and therefore I believe we are programmed for this. Our bad genes that get triggered from stressors that lead to disease get turned off. Our microbiome (gut bacteria) that is responsible for 70 percent of our immune system resets and becomes more diverse. All this leads to better health.

Keto Flex will teach you how to add this incredible concept to your daily life. Ben makes it so easy, and I predict you will not only experience an amazing breakthrough, but you will find that it is easier for you to stay on a healthy diet.

You are blessed to have this book in your hands.

Dr. Daniel Pompa, www.drpompa.com

Leading expert on cellular health

A respected leader in the health and wellness space, Dr. Pompa specializes in educating practitioners and the public on the origins of inflammation-driven disease, the therapeutic application of the ketogenic diet, fasting, ancestral-based health approaches, cellular healing, and detoxification.

Preface

On Tuesday, August 12, 2014, at noon, I received a phone call from the hospital.

Looking at the caller ID, my heart sank into my chest. I picked up the call and heard the words, "Mr. Azadi, your father stopped breathing this morning. We attempted to resuscitate him, but to no avail. He has passed away."

I sat down on my black leather couch, and a wave of emotions followed. Part of me was relieved that my father was no longer suffering, and the other part of me was devastated that I had lost him.

In the 1970s, my dad had immigrated to the United States with my mother. They made the bold decision to move to Miami Beach, Florida after my father was offered a job opportunity. They didn't speak a word of English. They learned by watching *Sesame Street*.

In 1980, my sister Sheila was born; and then on September 5, 1984, I was born.

My parents divorced when I was six years old. My father followed the Standard American Diet (SAD), and as a result he developed type 2 diabetes. I didn't understand the disease, and I blindly followed the instructions his conventional doctors gave him.

I remember driving my dad to his doctor's appointments and getting his insulin and blood sugar reducing medications. Every Tuesday, I took my dad to the grocery store to purchase the foods recommended by his doctor. I then proceeded to fill up his seven-day pill box for the week.

Year after year, my father's health declined. He gained weight and the dosage of his medications increased. One day he called me because he was having terrible diabetic neuropathy in his feet, and he was having a hard time walking. My mother and I picked him and took him to the emergency room. Neuropathy is when there's a lack of blood flow to the extremities caused by elevated sugar in the bloodstream. This can be a serious issue because it leads to infection, which could spread to the rest of the body and cause death. To prevent this from happening, doctors often amputate the feet in order to save the rest of the body. My father knew an amputation might be in his future. After being admitted to the emergency room, he experienced high amounts of stress thinking about the possibility of losing his feet. He ended up suffering a massive stroke, which left the entire right side of his body paralyzed, and he lost the ability to speak.

After the stroke, they transferred my dad to hospice care, where I would visit him each week. Week after week, I witnessed my father's body shrink before my eyes. Nine months into this extremely challenging time, I went to visit him. This was the evening of August 11. When I walked in the room, my father was in the worst shape I had ever seen. He was convulsing and throwing up on himself. I immediately flagged down the nurses to help. They cleaned him up, and he looked better. Before I left, I walked up to my dad and looked at him square in the eyes. His hopeless eyes looked back at me. I told him how much I loved him. I shared that he would always be my father and I would always be his son. I kissed him on the forehead and whispered the words "*hasta la vista,* baby." He always said that to me when he would say goodbye; he learned this from the movie *Terminator,* which was one of our favorites.

I drove home that night, sobbing the entire time. I remember getting home and praying. I said the same prayer I had been saying for weeks, which was to please end my father's suffering. It had been enough, and all I wanted was for him to be in peace. There was something different this time. I felt an energy, a feeling that someone, something, was listening to me. I went to bed, and twelve hours later I received that phone call about my father's passing.

Losing my father raised several questions for me. I wanted to know why my father had to go through so much pain when we had followed the advice from his doctors. It's not only my father—at least 60 percent of Americans are diabetic or prediabetic. Three out of four Americans are obese or overweight. Are we designed for sickness? Why is there such an epidemic of disease? I took a deep dive into the research, and to my surprise, I discovered that my father's doctors were only treating his *symptoms*. His doctors failed to see there was a *cause and an effect,* not just a result. I soon realized that the same information which I'm about to share with you in this book—the same information on stages all over the world—is the same information that could have saved my father's life. I also know that I was given that mountain so I can show the world this mountain can be moved. This is my pain-to-purpose message. This is why I've written *Keto Flex.*

If you are experiencing a symptom right now, that is actually not the problem; it is a result of the underlying disease.

You Cannot Drug Yourself to Perfect Health

Nobody dies from diabetes. They die from the degenerative diseases connected to it.

Here are the sickening statistics.

• 60 percent of Americans are diabetic or pre-diabetic

• 68 percent of these diabetics end up with heart disease

• 16 percent will have a stroke

• 70 percent end up with neuropathy where their nerves are degenerating

The above statistics apply to those who are on medication. Most people don't understand that just because you are taking medication, it doesn't mean you are exempt from this set of statistics.

Diabetes medication shows that the sugar levels may be getting better, but the diabetes is getting worse.

Conventional medicine treats the symptom (glucose), when the root cause is excessive insulin. By taking insulin, you are making the root cause worse and the diabetes worse. You can't superficially treat only the symptoms and expect the disease to get better. This is exactly what happened to my dad, and what's happening to millions of people.

With all due respect, when a doctor tells you your condition is terminal, what they should actually be saying is that their ability to help you is terminal.

Einstein said "Intellectuals solve problems; geniuses prevent them." You have in your hands the keys to the health kingdom. After reading this book, you will be empowered to understand that you are a genius. I believe you are a masterpiece because you are a piece of the master.

Did you know that you have 24/7 access to the world's greatest physician and healer? This inner physician is called the innate intelligence. The innate intelligence is designed to help your body heal. My goal with this book is to help you in three ways:

1. Identify interference.

2. Remove the interference.

3. Allow your body to heal.

When you remove the cause, the symptoms go away by default.

For example, I was obese the majority of my life. Growing up in Miami Beach, Florida, I followed the Standard American Diet. I was addicted to video games, drugs, and a toxic environment. Back in 2008, at the age of 24, I weighed 250 pounds. I was going through a tough break up with my girlfriend. I was depressed and looking for ways to end my life. Every time I explored suicide, I immediately thought of my mother, my family, and the devastation they would deal with if I took my own life. I was treating my health casually, and I believe when you treat your health *casually* you will end up a *casualty*.

For the first time in my life, I started to read books from incredible authors such as Bob Proctor, Wayne Dyer, Earl Nightingale, Zig Ziglar, Jim Rohn, and others. What these books helped me understand was that *I was responsible for my results*. Up until that point, I was blaming everyone else for my circumstances. Then I took ownership over my health. It's almost impossible to feel frustrated and upset when you take responsibility. Your ability to respond to life is responsibility.

I immediately stopped being the *victim of my past* and became the *victor of my future*.

I started to focus on my health, because the bigger the vision, the more energy is required to accomplish it. Fast-forward nine months, and I went from 250 pounds to 170 pounds, 34 percent body fat to 6 percent, size 38 waist to size 30. I finally carved out a physical six-pack, which was a dream since I was a young boy being bullied and made fun of for being overweight. But most importantly, I achieved a mental six-pack. I started to think better thoughts. I was no longer depressed and suicidal. No longer addicted to sugar, video games, and toxic people. The average person has 60,000 thoughts per day, and to think better thoughts brings tremendous rewards.

I learned that you don't get what you *want* in life, you get what you *are*; and what you are is your thoughts.

I changed my thoughts, and I changed my life. Wayne Dyer said, "When you change the way you look at things, the things you look at change."

This was a turning point for me, because it started my journey in the health space as a personal trainer, which evolved to becoming a CrossFit gym owner, and then to eventually getting a functional health practitioner certification with FDN.

The reason I share this with you is because I never had a weight *problem*, I had a weight *symptom*. When I took care of the cause, the effect went away by default. This book you have in your hands will help you identify the cause so that you can remove it and heal. I'm very excited for you! You are about to discover my 4 Pillars to doing so. In less than 60 days, you'll be able to reset your fat burning hormones and your biological clock to make disappear the many symptoms you're experiencing.

I'm very passionate about delivering this information to you so that you understand it and apply it. I built an online program called The Keto Kamp Academy which brings together a supportive community environment where I teach the tools necessary to help people overcome their symptoms and address the root cause. This book is a summary of my findings, and it will help you understand how incredible your self-healing body is.

Introduction

This book can transform your life.

Well, to a point. It can't make you rich or turn you into a celebrity—you'll have to get those on your own.

But it can do something just as valuable. Perhaps even *more* valuable.

It can make you happy with yourself. It can help you have more energy, feel better, and enjoy better health. It can give you a new, positive outlook on life, and help you to wake up each morning ready to conquer the world.

And to accomplish these wonderful things, you don't have to do a darn thing other than *eat.*

Crazy, right?

Of course, it all depends on *what* you eat and *when* you eat it.

This book is will show you how the familiar mix of everyday nutrients—protein, fat, and carbohydrates—can change, and by changing, will make a big difference in your health. You'll see how cutting carbs and consuming more fat and protein will change the way your body creates the energy it needs to live and thrive.

I can hear the sound of brakes screeching. "Stop!" you say. "You actually want me to eat *more fat?*"

Yes. The book will reveal how healthy fats have been maligned by the processed foods industry, which wants you to consume sugar, corn syrup, and artificial sweeteners, which *really are* bad for you. In fact, healthy fats such as nuts, olive oil, avocados, eggs, beef, and much more, can provide satiation and nutrition while allowing your body to shift from burning glucose—a sugar—to making molecules called ketones, which it can also use for energy. Your body makes ketones from the fat cells you already have (probably in abundance!). These fat cells are nature's ancient source of free energy for your body. They are waiting to be accessed, which will happen when certain conditions are met.

The key is not only *what* you eat but also *when* you eat. Thousands of years ago, our ancestors were accustomed to having sporadic supplies of food. They didn't always eat three meals a day. To them, this was normal, and the human digestive system was designed to function optimally with long periods between meals. The book will show you how to replicate those ancient conditions—which your digestive system will embrace —with deliberate, intermittent fasting. This dietary "flex" kickstarts the process of ketone production and puts you on the road to shedding excess fat, feeling good about yourself, and enjoying better health.

To make your Keto Flex lifestyle super easy, the book includes delicious fat burning menus, recipes, and shopping lists. All you have to do is stay focused on the positive outcome, and before you know it, your friends and colleagues will say, "Wow, you look terrific! What's the secret?"

Go ahead—tell them. They'll thank you for it!

Ready to transform your life? Let's get started!

Chapter 1: From Despair to Hope

Your life should be long and rewarding. It should be full of joy and excitement. The future should be bright, with every day bringing nothing but wonderment and gratitude.

The food you eat should give you energy and keep your mind and body healthy.

You should look forward to being happy and active on the day when you blow out one hundred candles on your birthday cake.

Take a moment and be honest: Is this your experience? Do you share these feelings?

If you're like millions of Americans, you're shaking your head and thinking, "My life, long and rewarding? Full of joy and excitement? Fat chance! My life is a grind. I wake up tired and go to sleep with heartburn. My doctor says I need to lose weight. Eating makes me happy—but only for a few minutes, and then I feel lousy again. Live to the age of one hundred? Hah! Dream on. I'll be bedridden by the time I'm ready to collect Social Security."

Sadly, in the wealthiest nation in the world, where we have every opportunity to achieve health, longevity, and personal happiness, too many people are sick. They are emotionally and physically sick. They are not as fulfilled as they could be, and they're not living as long as they should. I was in this exact position for the first 24 years of my life. I was mentally and physically bankrupt. My goals were the size of a pregnant ant, as I tiptoed my way through life hoping to land safely at death's door.

You've heard the statistics, but they deserve another look. As the Centers for Disease Control and Prevention (CDC) reported, in 2017-2018 the prevalence of obesity among U.S. adults was a whopping 36.5 percent. Another 32.5 percent of American adults are overweight. In all, more than two-thirds of adults in the United States are overweight or obese. Why does this matter? Because excess weight impacts health. Conditions directly related to obesity include type 2 diabetes, stroke, heart disease, and certain types of cancer. These chronic "lifestyle diseases" are some of the leading causes of premature, preventable death.

Obesity is expensive, too. In 2008, the estimated annual medical cost of obesity in the United States was $147 billion, and the medical cost for people who have obesity was $1,429 higher than those of healthy weight.

The average cost of treating a patient with type 2 diabetes is $14,000 per year.

The rise in obesity and diabetes is no accident. There is a clear cause: we're eating more food than ever before in human history. The average American consumes more than 3,600 calories daily, representing a 24 percent increase from 1961, when the average was just 2,880 calories per day. How many calories do scientists say we need to survive and be healthy? Daily intake should be around 2,500 for men and 2,000 calories for women. This means we're consuming, on average, about *40 percent more calories per day* than we need to be healthy and well nourished. These extra calories include a lot more processed carbohydrate. We're also eating more vegetable and seed oil, sugar, artificial sweeteners, alcohol, and grains including barley, wheat, rice, rye, maize, and cereal.[1]

Calorie *intake* is not the only measure of calorie *requirements*. We've all heard about the phenomenal calorie requirements of top athletes. During training for the Olympics, US swimmers Ryan Lochte and Michael Phelps consumed up to 8,000 calories every day. The size of their meals was legendary—for breakfast, Phelps reported eating three fried-egg sandwiches with cheese, lettuce, tomatoes, fried onions, and mayonnaise. Two cups of coffee. One five-egg omelet. One bowl of grain. Three slices of French toast topped. Three chocolate-chip pancakes.

---

[1] https://www.businessinsider.com/daily-calories-americans-eat-increase-2016-07#daily-calories-from-sugar-and-artificial-sweeteners-has-also-risen-by-almost-100-3

Australian swimmer Melanie Schlanger remarked that one of the best things about the Games was eating as much as she liked at the 24-hour McDonald's onsite at the Olympics.[2]

In reality, the vast majority of Americans are not top athletes, or even vaguely athletic. In fact, we're not only eating more, but we're moving less than we used to. Thanks to our computers, we are increasingly sedentary. Most Americans spend at least two hours a day watching television or videos, and we devote more time—both work and leisure—to sitting and staring at computer screens. Our inactivity comes at a price: Too much time spent sitting can increase a person's risk for diabetes, heart disease, and early death. It's often said the solution for this is to simply "eat less and move more." You'll learn later in the book why this is a flawed approach, and the actual cause of weight gain.

And heartburn! Over the past few decades, sales of heartburn medications have skyrocketed, and in 2020 the global market for gastroesophageal reflux disease (GERD) therapeutics reached $4.6 billion. Why? The primary cause of GERD is eating frequent large meals, which puts pressure on the lower esophageal sphincter (LES) muscle, allowing stomach acid to flow up into the esophagus and causing a burning pain in the chest. When empty,

---

[2] Quartz. https://qz.com/753956/how-olympic-swimmers-can-keep-eating-such-insane-quantities-of-food/#:~:text=Though%20Phelps%20later%20admitted%20the,the%20intensity%20of%20their%20workouts.

your stomach is only about the size of your fist, and as you'll learn later in the book, people who practice intermittent fasting very rarely experience heartburn.

Ironically, our increasingly sedentary lifestyle does not mean we're getting more quality sleep time—in fact, most of us get too little sleep. According to the CDC, more than a third of American adults don't get enough sleep on a regular basis, defined as an average of seven hours per night of uninterrupted snoozing. Sleeping less than seven hours per day is associated with an increased risk of developing chronic conditions including heart disease, diabetes, obesity, stroke, high blood pressure, and frequent mental distress. Why don't we sleep enough? Three big reasons: obesity increases sleep apnea, we have too many electronic devices keeping us awake, and shift work disrupts our natural circadian rhythms.

Medications can disrupt sleep too. As a society, we are increasingly medicated, with the average adult filling—get ready— more than 17 prescriptions every year. According to AARP, on average, people age 45 and older say they take four prescription medications every day. Many common medications can interfere with sleep. Those for high blood pressure and asthma can keep you awake all night with insomnia, while others including cough, cold, and flu medications can disrupt sleep. Other medications, such as antihistamines, can cause daytime drowsiness.

We are suffering not just physically, but emotionally. A study by Blue Cross and Blue Shield revealed that major depression is on the rise among Americans. It's happening in all age groups, but particularly among teens and young adults. The CDC reported that suicides are becoming more common in every age group, and especially among middle-aged people. Is there a link to the foods we eat? Apparently so. Researchers in China have found that a poor diet affects mental health, and that people who consume a diet high in processed meat, refined grains, sweets, potatoes, and gravy, along with low intakes of fruits and vegetables are at greater risk of depression.[3]

We aren't living as long as we should. After centuries of steadily increasing lifespans, life expectancy in the United States actually declined from 78.9 years in 2014 to 78.7 years in 2015, and then down to 78.6 years in 2017. We lag behind other comparable nations, who average a lifespan of 82.3 years. Leigh Erin Connealy, MD, shared on The Keto Kamp Podcast that in United States alone, 50 percent of the population is suffering from a chronic illness. The United States ranks 43rd in the world in chronic illness, which means many developing nations are doing better than us!

---

[3] https://www.sciencedirect.com/science/article/abs/pii/S0165178117301981#!

We are failing in biological life. One in four women are infertile, as are one in three males. As a species, we are literally losing the ability to procreate. We have other examples of species that had this problem and ended up becoming extinct.

According to the CDC, 1 out of 3 women and 1 out of 2 men are diagnosed with cancer during their lifetime. It's estimated by the year 2032, that 1 out of 2 children will be born on the autistic spectrum.

We know we're going in the wrong direction, and yet we struggle to find solutions. As we'll see in the pages ahead, despite the dire state we're in now, there's hope—but we need to make the right choices.

The George Costanza Effect

In our efforts to regain or achieve good health, we too often fall into what I call the George Costanza Effect. I first heard of this analogy from my colleague Dr. Jason Fung. It's named in honor of the *Seinfeld* TV show character, George, who has been described as neurotic and self-loathing, yet also prone to episodes of overconfidence that invariably arise at the worst possible times. He always manages to see a problem and then pursue the wrong solution, thereby making matters worse.

Americans can often correctly identify a problem, which is the first step towards healing. After all, when you see a doctor, his or her primary task is to properly diagnose your illness. Without a proper diagnosis, the cure will be misguided. Unfortunately, most conventional doctors diagnose the symptom, which can be far removed from the cause.

But having identified the problem, like George Costanza, too often we seek the wrong solutions and fall for half-baked theories and diets. On one of the episodes of *Seinfeld*, George had an idea to do the opposite of everything he had learned.

For example, when sitting down at a restaurant, he would always order a chicken salad, so instead he ordered a tuna salad. Then George walked up to a woman sitting alone, and instead of lying about who he was, he did the opposite and said, "My name is George. I live with my parents, and I'm bald." Remarkably, this was received well by the woman. Everything in George's life started to improve once he started doing the exact opposite of what he had been taught.

When we follow the exact opposite advice (the George Costanza Effect) of what the government promotes as a nutritional guideline, mainstream media endorses, and article headlines on your social media feed say, we end up getting better results in life.

What if I told you the same diet the American Diabetes Association website promotes is the exact diet that will lead to the development of diabetes?

What if I told you the food given to patients inside of the hospital going through chemotherapy, is the exact foods which can lead to cancer growth inside of the body?

This book will challenge your current way of thinking. It will go against conventional wisdom. I do not want you to believe anything written here. I do want you to have the faith to research and apply this information.

Take the issue of weight, and our collective recognition that many of us need to shed excess pounds. The American diet industry is huge. As PRNewswire reported, in 2020 the weight loss market was worth a whopping $71 billion. As many as 24 percent of American men and 40 percent of American women are actively dieting to lose weight, and according to a national telephone survey, 57 percent of U.S. women are dieting at any given time.

The weight loss industry is made up not only of companies developing diet plans and selling pre-packaged meals, but also weight-loss supplement manufactures, diet experts and obesity doctors, low-fat food makers, and low-calorie soda makers. Yes, there's even a SlimFast Keto line of products. Sigh.

Meanwhile, do-it-yourself plans abound as consumers use free diet and fitness apps. While the focus of the consumer is moving away from calorie counting and traditional "dieting" to a sustainable, healthier lifestyle, the fact remains that too many people are obese and overweight, and what they are doing, no matter how well intentioned, isn't working.

People are also getting mixed messages about weight. The fat acceptance movement strives to normalize obesity, which is understandable when you consider the scorn that has traditionally been heaped upon overweight and obese people by their slender peers. Fat activists assert that aggressive diet promotion and fat shaming have created an increase in psychological and physiological problems among overweight people. They argue that our culture's focus on weight loss is nothing more than the use of science to control deviance, and that the health challenges of being overweight or obese have been misrepresented or exaggerated and are used as an excuse for cultural and aesthetic prejudices against large people.

In the medical world, psychologists who are unhappy with the treatment of fat people have initiated the Health at Every Size movement, which has five basic tenets:

1. Enhancing health

2. Size and self-acceptance

3. The pleasure of eating well

4. The joy of movement

5. An end to weight bias

There is no doubt that your *mental* health influences and guides your *physical* health. If you are a large person and you are radiantly, sincerely, and truly happy, then you are likelier to be healthier than a person who desperately tries to lose weight and cannot. Is it better to be fat and happy than skinny and miserable? Perhaps, but even if you are indeed happy the stress that excess weight puts on your body is very real. For example, your hips and knees will give out more quickly. Obesity results in the necessity for the earlier replacement of knees and hips. For hip replacements, it's 10 years earlier than the general population, while for knee replacements, it's 13 years earlier. Costs tend to be higher, and after surgery, morbidly obese patients often experience more complications related to surgery and significantly more complications related to the wound.

If you have repeatedly tried and failed to lose weight, there is a small likelihood that your obesity has a genetic component. The CDC reports that genome-wide association studies have found more than 50 genes associated with obesity, most with minor effects. Most obesity is multifactorial—that is, caused by complex interactions among many genes and environmental factors. Genes may load the gun, but you decide to pull the trigger.

In her study, "Obesity, Epigenetics, and Gene Regulation," Jill U. Adams, Ph.D., showed the power of gene regulation in a family of agouti mice, in which genetically identical siblings looked entirely different in both color and size. She demonstrated that one mouse may be obese and yellow, but her twin sister may be small and brown. Yet another genetically identical sister may have a mottled look with both fur colors present and fall in the middle of the weight range.

How was this possible? While the genome of each of these mice was identical, the *gene expression* in each was quite different. It's simply a matter of which genes are "turned on" and which are kept "off."[4]

The bottom line is that even if your weight problem has a genetic component, you can still learn to eat a healthy diet, which is the subject of this book.

Get Healthy to Lose Weight

Weight loss is big business for four reasons:

1. Many people want to lose weight.

_____

[4] Nature.com. https://www.nature.com/scitable/topicpage/obesity-epigenetics-and-gene-regulation-927/

2. They sign up for expensive weight loss programs.

3. The weight loss programs fail.

4. They repeat the process over and over again.

The problem is that most programs, and even doctors, dietitians, and nutritionists, promote *losing weight to get healthy*.

This is not how the body works.

We don't lose weight to get healthy; *we get healthy to lose weight*.

The "lose weight to get healthy" approach creates a vicious cycle. A person gets on the scale and says, "I need to lose fifty pounds." They sign up for one of dozens of diet plans. They do the plan and lose some weight. But the plan is painful, and after a while they give up and go back to their old habits. The weight comes back. They get on the scale and say, "I need to lose fifty pounds—again." So, they sign up for another diet. Round and round it goes, like *Groundhog Day,* but without the happy ending.

Part of the problem is that the mechanisms of weight control are very complicated and susceptible to wild theories. This lack of understanding leads to the proliferation of solutions to nutrition and weight loss that don't lead to positive outcomes. Here are just three of the myths that mislead people who are trying to eat a healthy diet.

Myth #1: Calories in Vs Calories Out

It sounds logical, doesn't it?

This concept is based on the idea that as long as you consume fewer calories than you burn, you're bound to lose weight.

The problem is that it's much too simplistic and does not take into account real-life conditions.

For example, one cup of sugar contains 773 calories. Therefore, if you were to adhere strictly to the "calories in, calories out" formula, to reach your daily average adult female recommendation of 2,000 calories, all you would need to do is mix 2 ½ cups of sucrose (ordinary table sugar) in some water and drink it down. Voilà—you've just consumed exactly the number of calories you need per day to achieve a normal weight!

Of course, any sane person would say, "That's crazy! No one can live on sugar water! It's pure carbohydrate, with zero protein, zero fat, and zero trace minerals. If you ate nothing but sugar, you'd get sick and eventually die of malnutrition."

Yes, that is true. A sugar diet would kill you. In addition, as you headed towards death you'd suffer from horrible hyperglycemia and a host of other bad side effects.

The fact is that in terms of their effects on the human body, not all calories are *processed* equally. They come "packaged" in different foods, and how these foods are digested makes a huge difference in both how the calories are absorbed and how much they satiate your appetite. For example, consider 350 calories in an 8-ounce steak versus 350 calories in sucrose (table sugar):

One 8-ounce steak contains:

Calories: 350

Fat: 10 to 16 grams

Protein: 40 to 45 grams

Carbohydrates: zero

Minerals: iron, potassium, calcium.

In contrast, 350 calories of sucrose contain:

Calories (from carbohydrate): 350

Protein: zero

Fiber: zero

Vitamins and minerals: zero

This means that the calories from sucrose are instantly digested, converted into glucose, and absorbed into your bloodstream, causing your blood sugar level to spike sharply. Your brain receives a huge surge of a feel-good chemical called dopamine. Then when your blood sugar levels drop as your cells absorb the glucose, you may feel jittery and anxious—the "sugar crash." Prolonged consumption of sugar has been linked to a greater risk of depression.

But hey, it's just 350 calories, right?

In contrast, when you eat a steak, your digestive system has to work to free the 350 calories locked in the proteins and fat. The calories are released and introduced into your bloodstream slowly, over time. This keeps your blood sugar level stable, and the fat keeps you feeling full and satiated.

The fact is that getting too many of your calories from carbohydrates is unhealthy—but that's exactly what too many Americans do. In relation to overall caloric intake, carbohydrates comprise around 55 percent of the typical American diet, ranging from 200 to 350 grams per day. The vast potential of refined carbohydrates to cause harmful effects was relatively neglected until recently. A greater intake of sugar-laden food is associated with a 44 percent increased prevalence of metabolic syndrome and obesity and a 26 percent increase in the risk of developing diabetes mellitus.

The key concept to remember—which we will return to many times in this book—is that over the past 2.5 million years of human evolution, this is the way your digestive system was designed to work. Until very recently—really, just the past fifty years or so—

the human digestive system was accustomed to a diet high in natural fats, fiber, protein, and little carbohydrate. This was the nutrient mix it successfully utilized. Sugars—fructose from fruit, mainly—were bound up in fiber, and took a long time to extract.

Just to be clear, I'm not saying that the old days were some sort of utopia. Far from it. Life was short and starvation was not uncommon. Food shortages have been a feature of human life for millennia; the first famine in recorded history was during the reign of the Roman emperor Claudius, around 47 CE, which Luke cited in the book of Acts and the 4th century historian Orosius mentioned in the *Anglo-Saxon Chronicle*. Since then, famines have been regular occurrences, killing millions of people, with the most recent being in Yemen and South Sudan, which are occurring now. The point is that while starvation is bad, in our modern industrialized world, where *we can eat any way we choose*, it is incumbent upon us to be smart and not let the pendulum swing too far in the other direction. In developed nations, most of us can eat anything we want, whenever we want, and as much as we want. When we choose to indulge our appetites to the maximum, we make ourselves sick. That's just a fact.

Myth #2: Cholesterol and Saturated Fats Are Bad for You

This is another myth, promoted in the 20th century. It may have had its beginning with the modern emphasis on "slimming" that began in the 1920s. People knew about calories, and "counting calories" became the trendy thing to do. Because dieters knew that fat grams had nine calories each, whereas protein and carbohydrate grams had only four, "low calorie" became synonymous with "low fat." Plus, there was a neat symmetry to the language: if you want to shrink the fat cells in your body, what better place to start than by eliminating the fat in your diet? The words were synonymous. It seemed like an obvious conclusion.

In the 1960s, scientific studies purported to demonstrate a link between blood cholesterol, dietary fat, and heart disease. Research published in the Journal of the American Medical Association's *JAMA Internal Medicine* found that *the sugar industry* had paid for studies that downplayed the connection between sugars and heart disease. Instead, these studies implicated fat as the main cause of heart disease—leaving out the fact that sugar is a major culprit. The scam worked brilliantly. As NBC News reported, Cristin Kearns, a University of California San Francisco researcher who is focusing on the sugar industry said, "by the 1980's, few scientists believed that added sugars played a significant role in coronary heart disease, and the first 1980 Dietary Guidelines for Americans focused on reducing total fat, saturated fat, and dietary cholesterol for coronary heart disease prevention." Stanton Glantz of the

University of California San Francisco's Center for Tobacco Control Research and Education added, "These tactics are strikingly similar to what we saw in the tobacco industry in the same era."[5]

Almost overnight, food manufacturers rushed to produce "low-fat" versions of nearly every conceivable type of processed food, from milk to baked goods. The problem was that to give these bland products flavor, they started adding more sugar and high-fructose corn syrup, which *really are* bad for you and promote obesity. Our obsession with low-fat foods continues to this day, even though the scientific evidence that is piling up proves the entire "fat scare" of the past fifty years has been dangerous nonsense. Educated people are turning back to food products like real butter and red meat because they are healthier and keep you more satiated than their low-fat versions, and that good feeling of satiation is key in weight control.

The "villain" of the stories, cholesterol, is a waxy substance that's a vital part of the membrane structure of every cell in your body. Your body also needs it to make hormones and vitamin D, among other important functions. In short, cholesterol is necessary for human life. If you had no cholesterol in your blood, you would die.

---

[5] NBC News. https://www.nbcnews.com/health/health-news/sugar-industry-manipulated-heart-studies-review-finds-n646836

Cholesterol is made by your liver and also comes from foods derived from animals, such as meat, full-fat dairy products, and poultry. Some tropical oils, such as palm and coconut oil, can also cause your liver to produce more cholesterol.

The science of cholesterol is evolving. Since the 1960s, we've been told the dietary cholesterol in foods raises blood cholesterol levels and causes heart disease, and that cholesterol is bad. While 50 years ago this conclusion may have been understandable based on the available science, better, more recent evidence doesn't support it. And the supposed problem isn't even the cholesterol itself. Lipoproteins are particles that transport cholesterol molecules in the bloodstream around your body. A high level of LDL lipoproteins has been associated with a greater risk of heart disease, whereas a high level of HDL lipoproteins actually lowers your risk.

This may surprise you, but research has shown more people die with heart disease with normal to low cholesterol than high cholesterol. A 2009 study from the University of California, Los Angeles, revealed that nearly 75 percent of patients hospitalized for a heart attack had cholesterol levels that would indicate they were *not* at high risk for a cardiovascular event, based on current national cholesterol guidelines.[6]

---

[6] ScienceDaily. https://www.sciencedaily.com/releases/ 2009/01/090112130653.htm

Confused? If so, you have plenty of company in the scientific community. The bottom line is that consuming moderate amounts of quality fat, as humans have done for millions of years, is one of the keys to good health.

Myth #3: Eat Lots of Small Meals All Day

As we'll discuss later in the book, how *often* we eat is just as important as *what* we eat.

For most of human history, food was available only intermittently during the day. When you were working in the fields, you couldn't stop for a "snack." You filled your belly at mealtime, worked for many hours, and then took another meal. It was common for healthy people to go without food for 12 hours or more at a time—typically from dinner until breakfast the next day. Food had to be rationed, especially during the winter, when your precious supply of carbohydrates (grains, mostly) could not be replenished until the next harvest. There was nothing unusual about this; it was just the normal routine. There were no refrigerators stocked with fresh food, no Taco Bell open at midnight, no 24-hour restaurants. When the sun went down, your outside labor ceased, and you rested until dawn.

Despite millions of years of our success living on earth, today we see many health "gurus," nutritionists, and dietitians advising people to portion control, cut calories, and eat every two or three hours. They say this strategy of "grazing" will help you lose weight and keep your metabolism "revved up."

Are they right? Somewhat yes, but mostly no. In the short term, this may appear to work, but in the long term it has a 99 percent failure rate.

Here's just one problem with grazing: If you want to age faster than anyone else in your neighborhood, then eat every two or three hours.

Why does this happen?

Because of cell duplication. When you are constantly giving yourself calories, your body starts to duplicate its cells. This is great for a growing child, but bad for a grown adult. Accelerated cell division is the essence of aging. You can test this by getting blood work. The markers to look at are your triglyceride-to-HDL ratio (1:1 is optimal, while over 3.5-to-1 could be dangerous), inflammatory markers like C-reactive protein and homocysteine, and metabolic markers like fasting blood glucose and fasting blood insulin.

Furthermore, many diseases start in the gut. Healthy gut, healthy you. If you're grazing and constantly have food in your stomach, you're not allowing your digestive system to rest.

Some of the major contributors to digestive disorders such as heartburn, indigestion, and food intolerance are underlying metabolic problems including lack of enzymes, intolerance to foods, chemical toxicity, and chronic constipation. Many of these symptoms are caused by eating too frequently. Eating meals too often does not allow the body enough time to recuperate between meals and reload its enzyme pool. This can cause a lack of enzymes and hydrochloric acid in the stomach, leading to the development of digestive disorders with conditions such as acid reflux (heartburn), esophageal disorders, and food intolerance.[7]

A fascinating study was done at the University of Virginia. Researchers took a group of college students and fed them 800 calories of Mellow Mushroom pizza and tracked how much stress this meal caused within the digestive tract.

Keep in mind that younger people typically have a faster digestive system.

What they discovered was astounding.

Fourteen hours after eating, this meal was *not* fully digested!

Dr. Bush explained on The Keto Kamp Podcast when you eat 2 or 3 meals per day with these processed high-carbohydrate meals (typical SAD fare); it destroys the gut integrity, at the tight junction's level. This leads to leaky gut, and overall dysfunction of the intestinal lining.

----

[7] Ori Hofmekler, the *Anti-Estrogenic Diet*, page 110.

What happens next? The liver gets inflamed, and then changes the hormonal cascade.

The liver dictates the endocrine system in a huge way. When you stress the liver, it can develop fatty liver very quickly. Inflammatory genes cascade through the entire system, the blood brain barrier breaks down, kidney tubules stop filtering well, and you become a sponge for toxins and inflammation.

Chronic digestive stress leads to digestive and autoimmune disorders. You can get stuck as a "sugar burner."

When you use fat as the primary fuel source, it burns very clean, as opposed to burning sugar, which is a "dirty" fuel source. Glucose burns quickly and easily, but it also burns dirty via excessive production of free radicals. Think of burning fat as a natural gas stove and burning sugar (glucose) as burning firewood. The gas stove burns very clean with no smoke; the firewood creates massive amounts of toxic smoke.

These are highly unstable molecules with one or more unpaired electrons in their outer shells. Free radicals are formed from molecules via the breakage of a chemical bond, such that each fragment keeps one electron. They are produced either from normal cell metabolisms or from external sources including radiation, pollution, medication, and cigarette smoke. Since they can be either harmful or helpful to the body, they play a dual role as both toxic and beneficial compounds. But when an excess of free radicals cannot be removed, their accumulation in the body generates a phenomenon called oxidative stress. Excessive free radicals are the driving force behind inflammation, cancer, and accelerated aging.

Therefore, grazing promotes the production of free radicals, which in excess are harmful and promote aging.

The secret to perfect health is in mimicking the eating behaviors of our hunter-gatherer ancestors. Science is showing that intermittent fasting enhances the body's resistance to oxidative stress and helps fight inflammation, another key driver of many common diseases.

In short, give your stomach a rest! Let it be empty for several hours a day, which is how it has worked for millions of years. This is the first step in going from bad health to good health, and from despair to hope.

Measuring Body Fat

This brings up two important questions: If we need *some* fat, then what's the right amount? And how do we measure body fat, anyway?

The second question is surprisingly difficult to answer. There are many ways to measure body fat, and they vary in accuracy and expense.

The Pinch Test

The simplest method is the pinch test, or the skinfold test. You can do it yourself, but if you use a pair of calipers, it's better if someone helps you. The idea is that if you pinch your flesh, the more subcutaneous fat you have, the thicker the pinch. Special skinfold calipers are used to measure the skinfold thickness in millimeters. Several measurements are recorded and averaged. Various skinfold testing protocols call for different measurement sites, but typically include the following seven locations on the body:

1. Abdomen - Next to the belly button

2. Suprailiac - Just above the iliac crest of the hip bone

3. Midaxillary - Midline of the side of the torso

4. Pectoral - The mid-chest, just forward of the armpit

5. Quadriceps - Middle of the upper thigh

6. Triceps - The back of the upper arm

7. Subscapular - Beneath the edge of the shoulder blade

Once you have taken skinfold measurements, you can go online to a website, and convert these numbers into a percent of body fat.

Other Methods

Body fat scales and body circumference measurements are methods you can do on your own.

Body fat scales look like regular bathroom scales. They work with the help of sensors underneath your feet that use bioelectrical impedance. When you step on the scale, a small electrical current runs up through your leg and across your pelvis, measuring the amount of resistance from body fat. You simply step on the scale, and the tool measures both your body weight and your estimated fat percentage.

Measuring your waistline can help complement your body fat scale results. The National Heart, Lung and Blood Institute advises that your risk for heart disease and diabetes increases if you are a woman with a waist measurement greater than 35 inches (88.9 cm) or a man with a waist measurement of more than 40 inches (101.6 cm).

Dual-energy x-ray absorptiometry (DEXA) scans are used to measure bone mass for osteoporosis diagnoses. They are also reliable methods of body fat measurement. To get one of these scans, you'll need to find a center that has the equipment and test, which is typically not covered by insurance and can be expensive.

MRI and CT scans are the most accurate methods of measuring body fat. However, these imaging tests are usually limited to medical research and are very expensive.

Underwater weight (hydro-densitometry) tests are based on the idea that fat is more buoyant than muscle. Until CT scans and MRI scans were developed, it was considered the gold standard for measuring body composition. During the test, your body is weighed on land and underwater. The difference between these two measurements allows test administrators to calculate your body density and body fat percentage. For example, let's say two men— Jim and Bob—have exactly the same weight on dry land. When submerged, Jim weighs *more* than Bob—that is to say, Bob is more buoyant. Therefore, Bob has proportionally more body fat.

Athletes use hydro densitometry to measure their body fat at different points during their season and monitor their fitness. They'll take a baseline reading at the beginning of the training year and retest at the end of each training block.

Body Fat Percentage

After all that measuring, let's get back to the first question: What's the result you want?

Here are the guidelines from the American Council on Exercise:

Percent Body Fat Norms for Men and Women

Gender	Women	Men
Minimum healthy level	10-13%	2-5%
Athletes	14-20%	6-13%
Fit people	21-24%	14-17%
Maximum acceptable	25-31%	18-24%
Obese	32% +	25% +

As you can see, there's a very definite minimum acceptable percentage of fat in your body: For men, its 2 percent, and for women it's 10 percent. Other sources put the minimum male body fat at 5 percent, with athletes occasionally dipping below. This is the number your primal brain is watching.

Why not go for zero fat?

Because fat cells perform many critical functions, without which you won't live very long.

• **Hormone production**. Fat cells make both estrogen and leptin, which are needed for puberty and reproduction. Low leptin levels can mean lowered testosterone levels. Insufficient leptin and testosterone levels can result in hypogonadotropic hypogonadism, or secondary hypogonadism, in which the reproductive system basically shuts down. In plain English, this means if you're a man, you'll have a new nickname: "Mr. Softee."

• **Brain health.** Fat is critical for brain function. For example, individuals with the eating disorder anorexia nervosa, who are characterized by self-starvation and minimal body fat, experience a decrease in brain size and volume. The health of your fat is directly connected to the health of your brain!

• **Immune system.** Leptin strengthens your immune system and assists in wound healing. Anorexics have weaker immune systems and heal slower than those with minimum fat levels. Low body fat and energy intake is also associated with higher cortisol levels, which hamper the immune system, increasing your risk of bacterial infection or contracting a cold or flu virus.

• **Heart health.** Having an extremely low body-fat percentage can affect the cardiovascular system's ability to function normally and can lower the heart rate. Abnormally low heart rates, called bradycardia, can lead to dizziness, passing out, and cardiac arrest.

• **Body heat.** Fat cells play a role in providing insulation for organs and helping the body maintain its temperature. People with extremely low body fat often feel cold all the time.

• **Hunger control.** Dieting down to minimal levels of body fat decreases circulating levels of leptin. Leptin receptors in the hypothalamus sense this drop and increase your appetite, so that you're constantly hungry.

The goal of fasting and reducing your percentage of excess body fat is to *enhance* your health, not *destroy* it with starvation!

Throw Away Your Bathroom Scale!

Why do I say this? Isn't measuring your weight important?

As a part of your overall health, your weight is important. But looking at the scale and then saying, "I need to lose weight because then I'll be healthier" is putting the cart before the horse. It's "back asswards," as they say. It's the opposite of what you want to do.

If you focus only on losing weight, you will be miserable, and you will probably fail. Here's a question worth pondering: Do you know why the weight loss industry in America is worth $2.6 billion dollars? It's because diet programs, where you enroll and eat the food they sell to you, have millions of *repeat customers*. They are repeat customers because traditional dieting, where the goal is to lose weight, fails. It fails *over and over again*. Sure, you may lose weight on a diet, but statistics prove that most people just gain back the pounds. So, then they need to go back on a diet. It's called "yo-yo dieting" for a good reason.

The reasons for yo-yo dieting are varied but often include embarking upon a calorie-restricted diet that's too extreme and focused on the wrong foods. At first the dieter experiences elation at the thought of weight loss and pride in their rejection of food.

But over time, the painful limits imposed by unnatural diets can cause depression or fatigue, making the diet impossible to sustain. The dieter inevitably reverts to his or her old eating habits, but now with the added psychological burden of having failed to lose weight by a restrictive diet.

In contrast, the Keto Flex lifestyle is focused on improving your *health*, beginning with your trillions of individual cells. The Keto Flex diet makes you feel good, not miserable. Many practitioners report a feeling of freedom the opposite of the restrictive feeling of hallmark traditional diets. You'll feel the difference in your energy level, your overall happiness, and the tone of your body. Will you lose weight? As you consume fat for energy, yes, you will. But that just goes along with the idea that if you correct an underlying condition, the symptoms—in this case excess body fat—will take care of themselves.

Chapter 2: Cellular Health, Energy, and Hormones

Your body is built of cells. There are many different types of cells with individual functions, but every cell consists of three basic parts: the cell membrane, the nucleus, and, between the two, the cytoplasm.

The cell membrane functions as the outer "skin" of the cell while controlling passage of materials into and out of the cell. It is composed of a double layer of phospholipid molecules. ("Lipid" means "fatty." Yep, there's that word again!) Proteins in the cell membrane provide various services including structural support and the formation of channels for passage of materials. Think of the cell membranes as the bodyguards of your cells.

The nucleus is the control center of the cell. It determines how the cell will function, as well as the basic structure of the cell. Threads of chromatin in the nucleus contain deoxyribonucleic acid (DNA), the genetic material of the cell. The nucleolus is a dense region of ribonucleic acid (RNA) in the nucleus.

Do you know how many cells form the average human body? No? Well, you're in good company. Scientists aren't certain.

According to an estimate published in 2013 in the *Annals of Human Biology* by an international team of researchers, and appropriately entitled "An estimation of the number of cells in the human body," it may be 37.2 trillion cells. It's just an educated guess.[8]

If lined up, our cells would wrap around the earth two million times. Our internal and external environments affect our cells. With the DNA we have, it gets injured throughout the day, every day, and we have to repair our genome several times a day.

According to Dr. Zach Bush's research, in just seconds the micro-RNA can adapt. A single gene can make over 200 different proteins. Who decides which genes are made? The micro-RNA governs it. With our 20,000 genes we can build 4 million different variants of ourselves. Those are a lot of options. When we're diagnosed with cancer or heart disease, we're not told that. We are told that this disease came upon us, and it's not our fault, it was "in our genes," or just bad luck.

What they never tell us is, "Hey, do you want to build yourself a new body?"

We can literally build new bodies. We've seen this many times before. When you run into an old high school friend who all of a sudden look completely different—well, they built themselves a different body. Five percent of the miRNA in our blood right now

[8] https://handling-solutions.eppendorf.com/cell-handling/about-cells-and-culture/detailview/news/how-many-cells-are-in-your-body-probably-more-than-you-think/

is from the food we eat (meat and plants). Fifteen percent is from the bacteria in our environment. Fifteen percent is from the fungi in our environment. We are what we ate. We are also what we ate's stress. If you have a conventional cow raised on a feeding lot, the stress of the cow will be transferred to the health of the human being who consumes it. We think this is happening mostly through the micro-RNA.

The cytoplasm is the gelatinous fluid that fills the cell. It provides support for the hundreds of organelles, which are the subcellular structures with specific jobs to perform in the cell, much like the organs in the body. All of the functions for cell expansion, growth, and replication are carried out in the cytoplasm of a cell. Within the cytoplasm, molecules (such as oxygen) move around by diffusion, which is the intermingling of substances by the natural movement of their particles.

Your brain, which runs the show, consists between 86 and 100 billion neurons, which are the specialized cells that "do the thinking" and create tiny electrical charges. In addition, there are about an equal number of glial cells that maintain homeostasis, form the fatty myelin insulation around the wire-like dendrites that connect the neurons (yet another example of the vital importance of fat), and provide support and protection for neurons.

The fuel that powers your brain is glucose and oxygen, which are via the bloodstream. Like other cells in the body, the respiration process in the brain cells creates waste or byproducts including carbon dioxide, water, ammonia, and various types of proteins. In the brain, two proteins in particular are produced: amyloid beta and tau. Amyloid beta is what forms the plaques found in the brains of Alzheimer's patients. Tau, which resembles sets of parallel railroad tracks, can be damaged or "tangled" and cause mitochondrial dysfunction. Tangles of tau are the hallmark of many neurodegenerative diseases.

Luckily, the brain has a mechanism to clear out tau and amyloid waste, called the glymphatic system, which scientists have dubbed the "garbage truck of the brain." The glymphatic system is activated during stage 4 delta sleep, where there is this dishwasher-like fluid which flushes over the brain as it temporarily shrinks and removes toxic waste.[9]

The Lifespan of a Cell

On a regular basis, the vast majority of the cells in your body die and are replaced by identical copies. You are literally not the

---

[9] https://www.sciencedaily.com/releases/2019/02/190227173111.htm

same person you were a few years ago. You look the same and may behave the same, but your actual cells are different.

Here's a good analogy. Everyone knows the U.S.S. *Constitution*, fondly called "Old Ironsides." This wooden warship was launched in 1797, and finally retired from active service in 1881. She's still a commissioned Navy vessel—the oldest ship to have that designation. At her berth at the old Charlestown Navy Yard in Boston, she's well cared for. As the decades have passed, the wooden parts have rotted, and the metal parts rusted or corroded. Periodically, the ship is dry-docked, and the damaged parts are replaced with identical new parts. This has been done so often that the ship is now estimated to be 85 percent replaced. Only 15 percent—mainly the massive keel of white oak—is original. Yet if a sailor from the 19th century were to be magically transported to the ship today, he'd be hard pressed to see the changes. For all practical purposes, Old Ironsides is the same ship she was back in 1797.

Your body is repaired and replaced in much the same way. In an adult, each day as many as 100 billion cells die and are replaced by other cells. The length of a cell's life varies depending on the type. For example, white blood cells live for about thirteen days, cells in the top layer of your skin live about 30 days, red blood cells live for about 120 days, and liver cells live about 18 months. Even your bones are replaced—osteocytes, which comprise up to 95 percent of the total bone cells, have a lifespan of no more than 25 years.

In contrast, brain cells are thought to last an entire lifetime—for example, scientists believe the neurons in the cerebral cortex are not replaced if and when they die. But brain cells that are damaged can often regenerate, in a process called neurogenesis.

The process of natural cell renewal is called *programmed cell death*. It plays a key role in balancing cell proliferation and maintaining constant cell numbers in the tissues, as well as being one of the first lines of defense against cancer and infection by invaders such as viruses.

You may be wondering about fat cells. Your body can make new ones, and the number of fat cells, or adipocytes, increases through childhood and adolescence, and then generally stabilizes in adulthood.

But adipocytes can change in size. Unlike most other types of cells, which cannot change their size, fat cells will expand and contract with weight gain or weight loss. And like most cell types in the body, adipocytes eventually die. Then they are replaced by new fat cells. Cell death and new cell production appear to be tightly coupled. About 10 percent of adipocytes die each year and are replaced at the same rate.

Beyond their role in storing fat, adipocytes secrete hormones and proteins that affect energy metabolism. Some scientists believe that while *losing* weight is relatively easy, it may be hard to *keep it off* because as adipocytes become smaller, they might send signals to increase appetite and fat storage.

To survive and thrive, every cell in your body must have a constant supply of vital substances including glucose, oxygen, and trace minerals, and they must be able to dispose of waste products including lactic acid, acetic acid, carbon dioxide, ammonia, and urea.

Glucose, Glycogen, and Ketones

Before we discuss the best strategies for maintaining optimal cell health, we need to learn about glucose, glycogen, and ketones.

If you study how the body transforms various molecules into energy for the body, you'll learn about a group of terms that are synonymous. The Krebs cycle, also known as the citric acid cycle (CAC) and the TCA cycle (tricarboxylic acid cycle), refers to the series of chemical reactions used by all aerobic organisms to release stored energy through the oxidation of acetyl-CoA derived from carbohydrates, fats, and proteins. In addition, the cycle provides precursors of certain amino acids, as well as the reducing agent NADH, which are used in numerous other reactions.

It's named after Hans A. Krebs, who, in 1937, first elucidated the process of cells converting food into energy, which he called the citric acid cycle. Krebs proposed a specific metabolic pathway within the cells to account for the oxidation of the basic components of food—carbohydrates, protein and fats—into energy. The Krebs cycle takes place inside the mitochondria or "power plants" of cells, and provides energy required for the organism to function.

In order to perform energy conversion, the mitochondria require oxygen, which is delivered to the cells by the respiratory and circulatory systems. The consumption of oxygen by mitochondria is called cellular respiration.

During times of food shortfall or fasting—even for short periods overnight—amino acids can be converted via the Krebs cycle to glucose for energy or for storage as glycogen and fat.

In healthy humans, the body continually makes a small amount of ketones to be used for energy. In times of fasting, and even overnight while sleeping on an empty stomach, the liver creates more ketones and the amount of ketone bodies in the blood increases.

Here's how the body converts various substances in fuel for its cells.

The normal pathways to create energy for the cells involve either stored carbohydrate or non-carbohydrate substances. Glycogen is a substance deposited in bodily tissues as a store of carbohydrates. Technically, it's a multibranched polysaccharide of glucose that serves as a form of energy storage in animals, fungi, and bacteria. "Polysaccharide" means "many sugars," and glycogen consists of a small central core to which more than ten molecules of glucose (sometimes there are dozens) are attached.

The conversion of glucose into glycogen is called *glycogen synthase*. Glycogen serves as an energy reserve that can be quickly mobilized to meet a sudden need for glucose. The controlled breakdown of glycogen and release of glucose increase the amount of glucose that is available between meals. Hence, glycogen serves as a buffer to maintain blood-glucose levels.

The process of converting glycogen back into glucose is *glycogenolysis*, in which glycogen stored in the liver and muscles is converted first to glucose-1- phosphate and then into glucose-6- phosphate, for use as energy by the cells. Glucagon from the pancreas and epinephrine from the adrenal glands are the two hormones that control glycogenolysis.

When ample carbohydrate stores are available, the main pathway for energy production is glycogenolysis, the breakdown of glycogen stores in muscle and liver. *Gluconeogenesis*, the production of glucose from non-carbohydrate sources such as lactate, is often utilized as well, especially in situations involving physical exercise.

A great analogy Dr. Jason Fung shared on The Keto Kamp Podcast is to think of your glycogen stores as the wallet you have inside of your purse or pocket. The cash inside of your wallet represents your glucose reserves. The benefit of using this source of energy is easy access. You can easily grab your wallet to pull cash out or put cash back in.

The drawback is that you have a limited capacity of how much cash you can store. Your glycogen stores are similar in that you can store about 2,000 calories in your glycogen stores. Anything more will be pushed into fat cells, leading to weight gain.

This might sound like a good option as the primary source of energy, but it is not. When you are relying on your sugar reserves for energy, you'd have to eat every few hours just to replenish your stores. Otherwise, your energy levels crash, and you end up feeling "hangry" (hungry and angry). Dave Asprey calls this "hypoglybitchy." It's not fun being a sugar burner.

Think of your fat stores as your bank safe. The drawback is that it takes longer to gain access to your bank safe verses your wallet. You have to drive to the bank and wait in line before you have access. The benefit is that there's unlimited reserves in your bank safe. This is the same case when it comes to your fat stores. You can store hundreds of thousands of calories of body fat on your body. For example, someone who has 10 percent body fat, which is very lean, has enough calories in the form of body fat to go several days without food and still survive. The goal here is to achieve the metabolic switch of burning through our glycogen stores (the wallet) so that our metabolism can start burning our fat cells (the bank safe).

When carbohydrate stores are significantly decreased, the liver makes up the shortfall through the upregulation of the ketogenic pathway and an increased production of ketone bodies.

How to Test Your Ketone Levels

There are three different methods for testing your ketone levels — blood, breath, and urine. Urine testing is only helpful in the beginning stages of keto-adaptation when your body is still learning how to use the ketones you're creating. During this time, a good portion of the ketone bodies acetoacetate you produce will get filtered out through your urine. This can give insight into whether or not your body is producing ketones. However, over time, your body will become more adapted, and the number of ketones lost in your urine will decrease.

Breath testing is a valid way to test the ketone bodies acetone, and is much less invasive than blood testing, but it may be less accurate. I have recently discovered an accurate breath ketone meter from BioSense. You can visit www.mybiosense.com to get their breath ketone meter. Use the coupon code ketokamp for $20 off.

The most common way to test ketones is with blood. I personally use the Keto Mojo device that tests for BHB in the blood.

Ketones (beta-hydroxybutyrate, or BHB) are water-soluble molecules produced by the liver from fatty acids during periods of low food intake, such as fasting and carbohydrate restrictive diets. Ketone bodies are readily transported into tissues outside the liver and converted into acetyl-CoA, a molecule that participates in many biochemical reactions in protein, carbohydrate, and lipid metabolism. These acetyl-CoA molecules enter the Krebs cycle and are oxidized in the mitochondria of each cell for energy. Ketone bodies can be utilized as fuel in the heart, brain, and muscles. In the brain, they are used to make acetyl-CoA into long-chain fatty acids.

Your level of ketones can be measured in your blood. The unit of measurement is the millimole. A mole is an amount of a substance that contains a large number (6 followed by 23 zeros) of molecules or atoms. Abbreviated "mmol," a millimole is one-thousandth of a mole. It's measured per liter of blood, as in "1.0 mmol/L."

If your ketogenic diet goal is weight loss, then 0.5 mmol/L to 1.0 mmol/L is a good starting point.

From there, aim for "optimal ketosis," which is when your ketone levels are between 1.0 mmol/L to 3.0 mmol/L. This is perfectly healthy and puts you in fat-burning mode.

People using the ketogenic diet for therapeutic benefits for medical conditions such as epilepsy, cancer, or endocrine and metabolic disorders, might aim for much higher ketone levels, in the 3.0 mmol/L to 5.0 mmol/L range.

Those who are fasting or consuming a much higher fat-to-protein ratio can post levels in the range of 3.0 mmol/L to 8.0 mmol/L. But you don't need to aim that high. The optimal ketosis range is called "optimal" for a reason, and it's ideal for weight-loss and general health purposes.

Here at Keto Kamp, we do not chase ketones. We chase *results*.

Ketogenesis is the metabolic pathway that produces ketone bodies, which provide an alternative form of energy for the body. The term is based on "keto" (ketone body) and "genesis" (birth). This essentially means your liver is producing ketones to fuel the body.

Burning fat and producing ketones is our primal birthright. Did you know that soon after babies are born, they enter a natural state of ketosis? Yep, you read that right—research shows that newborn infants are in ketosis and remain in this normal, healthy state while breastfeeding.

Furthermore, research confirms that breast milk from healthy mothers is actually made up of 50 to 60 percent fat, *and* the cholesterol in breast milk supplies babies with almost six times the amount that most adults consume in their diets. This helps the development of the baby's brain since it is made mostly of fat. God (or Mother Nature, if you prefer) doesn't make mistakes.[10]

Most organs and tissues can use ketone bodies as an alternative source of energy. During periods where glucose is not readily available, the brain uses them as a major source of energy. The heart typically uses fatty acids as its source of energy, but cal also use ketones.

---

[10] https://pubmed.ncbi.nlm.nih.gov/15573408/, https://pubmed.ncbi.nlm.nih.gov/15916931/, https://pubmed.ncbi.nlm.nih.gov/10652985/

Insulin regulates many key enzymes in the ketogenic pathway, and a state of low insulin triggers the process. A low insulin state leads to an increase in free fatty acids (FFAs), increased uptake of FFAs into the mitochondria of the cells, and increased production of ketone bodies.

Here's the bottom line, in plain English: Ketones are a form of fuel made by your liver. Your liver produces ketones when your blood is low on glucose, which your body ordinarily uses for energy, or you don't have enough insulin in your bloodstream to turn sugar into glucose. Because you always need energy for your brain and muscles, your liver then turns fat into ketones, a type of acid, and sends them into your bloodstream. Your brain, muscles, and other tissues can then use these ketones for fuel.

When ketones are produced faster than they can be used, they can be broken down into CO_2 and acetone. The acetone is removed by exhalation. One symptom of ketogenesis is that the person's breath smells sweet, like alcohol.

Can you have too many ketones in your blood? Yes. Just like you can have too much sugar in your blood (hyperglycemia), you can have too many ketones, a condition called *ketoacidosis*. It's most often associated with diabetes, called *diabetic ketoacidosis*. Signs of diabetic ketoacidosis include excessive thirst, frequent urination, nausea, vomiting, abdominal pain, shortness of breath, fruity-scented breath, and confusion. Among non-diabetic people, with moderate and controlled fasting, ketoacidosis is usually not a problem.

Hormones

The complex chemical activities of the body are controlled by the endocrine system and the central nervous system. The endocrine system does its part by secreting complex chemical substances called hormones into the blood stream. These secretions come from a variety of endocrine glands, which are special groups of cells. The major endocrine glands are the pituitary, pineal, thymus, thyroid, adrenal glands, and pancreas. In addition, men produce hormones in their testes and women produce them in their ovaries.

There are hundreds of hormones in your body. The key functions of hormones are to regulate the metabolic functions of the body (energy level, reproduction, growth and development, and response to injury, stress, and environmental factors); to regulate the rate of chemical reactions in various cells; and to influence the ability of substances to transport themselves through cell membranes.

Principle hormones include:

• Triiodothyronine (T3) and thyroxine (T4), which regulate weight and determine energy levels. T4 needs to be activated to T3 in order to be used by the cells.

• Insulin is released by the pancreas and moves glucose from the bloodstream into the cells; is the only fat storage hormone in the body.

• Serotonin, the mood-boosting hormone associated with learning and memory, regulating sleep, digestion, regulating mood, and some muscular functions.

• Cortisol, which helps you stay healthy and energetic. Its main role is to control physical and psychological stress. When you're in danger, it increases heart rate, blood pressure, respiration, and other "fight or flight" responses. It increases the metabolic rate, dilation of blood vessels going to the heart and the brain.

• Adrenaline is known as the "emergency hormone," because when danger or urgency are present, it initiates a quick reaction, making the person think and respond quickly to the stress. Adrenaline is secreted in the medulla in the adrenal gland, as well as some of the central nervous system's neurons.

• Growth hormone, also known as somatotropin hormone, is important in human development because it stimulates growth, cell reproduction, and cell regeneration, and boosts metabolism.

Because this book is focused on diet and nutrition, we'll focus on those hormones that impact those important areas.

Glucocorticoid Hormones

Your body has natural, daily cycles, called the circadian rhythm. Many functions—falling asleep at night, waking up, eating, and going to the bathroom—are patterned around a repeating 24-hour cycle. To prompt the body to do these things at the right time, hormones rise and fall at specified times of the day. When you go against these natural circadian rhythms, your health may suffer. Disrupted circadian rhythms have been linked to obesity, sleep disorders, depression, and other health problems.

For example, a group of steroid hormones known as glucocorticoid hormones are secreted on a 12-hour cycle. These hormones drive adipocyte (fat cell) production from precursors.

Disrupting this cycle is linked to obesity. Some people have diseases such as Cushing's disorder, or undergo steroid treatments, that result in boosted levels of these hormones in the body, and are also linked to obesity.

In addition to this natural daily rhythm, your body also secretes glucocorticoids during stressful situations. Immediately after a stressful event is experienced, there is a corticotropin-releasing-hormone (CRH)-mediated suppression of food intake. This diverts the body's resources away from the less important need to consume food and toward prioritizing fight, flight, or withdrawal behaviors. But then, as the stressful event fades into memory, the opposite happens: there is a glucocorticoid-mediated stimulation of hunger and eating behavior.

Glucocorticoids are effective suppressors of inflammation, and multiple immune-modulatory mechanisms involving leukocyte apoptosis, differentiation, and cytokine production have been described.

Estrogen, Progesterone, and Testosterone

Especially in women, hormone balance and weight regulation are closely linked, and even slight changes can significantly affect the metabolism and therefore your weight. One common issue is that as women age, certain key hormone levels decrease, making weight gain more likely. Later in the book, you'll discover how to follow a ketogenic and fasting approach custom to women who are at different stages of life (cycling, peri-menopausal, and post-menopausal).

Women who are experiencing perimenopause and menopause will see their estrogen levels drop. The body then looks for estrogen held in fat cells, which spurs the body to make more fat to make up for the estrogen shortfall.

Progesterone is an endogenous steroid involved in the menstrual cycle, pregnancy, and embryogenesis. It's produced mainly in the ovaries following ovulation each month. As women age, progesterone levels also decrease. With a progesterone deficit comes that puffy, bloated feeling that accompanies water retention.

Most people think of testosterone as a male sex hormone, but everyone requires a certain amount. While males have more testosterone than females, female adrenal glands and ovaries produce small amounts. In fact, women produce 20-30 times more testosterone than they do estrogen. Women lose testosterone during menopause, and because testosterone helps build muscle and burn calories, this hormone imbalance leads to muscle loss, lower metabolism, and weight gain.

Cortisol, Stress, and Belly Fat

Cortisol is one of the steroid hormones and is made in the adrenal glands. Cortisol helps regulate metabolism, control blood sugar levels, help reduce inflammation, and assist with memory formulation. It helps control blood pressure and has a stabilizing effect on salt and water balance.

Elevated levels of cortisol due to stress have been linked to weight gain, and particularly the accumulation of abdominal fat. Stress-induced abdominal fat is unhealthy because it secretes large amounts of inflammatory molecules that contribute to insulin resistance, diabetes, and heart attacks.

Insulin is the body's main hormone switch; it determines which fuel you will use—fat or sugar. If insulin is high, no fat will be burned—only sugar. If insulin is low, fat will be used exclusively as fuel.

Insulin has a bad public relations person, because it gets blamed for a lot of things. Insulin is actually a beautiful process that was designed by our creator; if we didn't have this process, humans wouldn't exist today.

When we eat carbohydrates, our bodies convert it into sugar (glucose), which raises blood sugar levels. The body then calls in the insulin troops to grab that sugar in the blood, and then insulin acts as a key to unlock your cells so that sugar can be moved into the trillions of cells.

If your blood sugar is normal, it means that you have roughly one teaspoon of dissolved sugar in your blood. An average person has about one gallon of blood in their body. So, you'd think that over the course of a day, you'd need very little sugar. But the average American consumes as much as 30 teaspoons of sugar every day. Faced with this high amount of ingested sugar, the body needs to bring the blood back to homeostasis (it's normal resting state), so anytime there's more than one teaspoon of sugar in the blood, insulin gets pumped into your blood to shuttle that glucose out of the blood and into your cells.

Just imagine how hard insulin has to work to remove this massively excessive amount of sugar from the blood! It has to work 30 times harder. That's insane.

Stress can also contribute to "middle-aged spread" because many sedentary people can't resist high carbohydrate foods—bread, doughnuts, cookies, cakes—to relieve their anxiety. In younger people, male and female hormones can protect against the deposition of abdominal fat, but after age 40, their levels start to decline.

Your body cannot distinguish between the stress produced by a lion chasing you and being stuck in a traffic jam. This is why it's imperative to master stress so that it is not chronically elevated leading to a host of symptoms. Stress is the silent killer that we all need to be aware of.

Ghrelin and Leptin

Our bodies have appetite- and weight-regulating hormonal mechanisms that strive to maintain hormonal homeostasis (that is, a steady hormonal "set point") throughout the day. When we take in less food energy than we expend through basal metabolism and activity, then our bodies respond by trying to correct the problem and make us hungry. Two vital hormones that modulate our appetite and hunger signals are ghrelin and leptin.

Ghrelin is a hormone that increases appetite and plays a role in body weight. I compare ghrelin to a gremlin, because it makes noise and it's not fun when it's around. Ghrelin causes you to pick up the fork. Ghrelin is released primarily in the lining of the stomach. It goes into the blood, crosses the blood-brain barrier, and arrives at your hypothalamus, where it tells you you're hungry. Researchers have suggested that ghrelin levels influence how quickly hunger comes back after you eat.

Leptin is a hormone secreted primarily in fat cells, as well as the stomach, heart, placenta, and skeletal muscle. It travels to the hypothalamus, and tells the hypothalamus that you have enough fat, so you can eat less or stop eating. It decreases your appetite. Leptin signals to your body to put down the fork. Leptin may also increase metabolism, although there is unresolved research on this point.

Leptin production correlates to fat mass—the more fat you have, the more leptin you produce. Levels of leptin are lower if you're a thin person, and higher if you're heavyset. So, you would think that having more leptin would help you lose weight, because it suppresses your appetite. The problem is that many obese people have built up a resistance to the appetite-suppressing effects of leptin.

Leptin resistance is similar to insulin resistance, and they share common signaling pathways. Insulin resistance occurs when there's plenty of insulin being produced, but the body and brain have stopped responding to its commands (type 2 diabetes). Once you arrive at a certain "fat mass," then your excess body fat will disrupt your appetite signals and actually make you hungrier.

Overall, research suggests that ghrelin production seems to be affected by growth hormone release, which differs in men and women. Leptin seems to influence fertility and reproduction in women, which are related to women's body fat levels. Women appear to be more sensitive than men to leptin levels. Dr Sylvia Tara's book *The Secret Life of Fat*, showed women produce 33% more ghrelin than men after exercise.

And above all, obesity can disrupt normal appetite signaling. In obese people, signals from leptin and ghrelin may not always work in the expected ways.

Sleep is a factor also. A lack of sleep results in less leptin and more ghrelin—which increases your appetite—as well as disrupted glucose and insulin metabolism. In addition, cortisol levels are higher when you do not get adequate sleep, which may also increase appetite. This can become a vicious cycle, which is why healthy sleep must be prioritized in order to maximize the Keto Flex lifestyle.

Research has shown repeatedly that poor sleep or inadequate sleep is linked to weight gain and a higher body mass index (BMI). While people's sleep requirements vary, short sleep duration increases the likelihood of obesity in both children and adults. Weight gain has been seen in experimental sleep deprivation studies, and the reward centers of the brain are more stimulated by food when you are sleep deprived. Poor sleep can increase the brain's pleasurable response to food and decrease your self-control and decision-making abilities.

To make the problem even worse, many sleep disorders, such as sleep apnea, are worsened by weight gain. It's a vicious cycle that can be difficult to break: Poor sleep can cause weight gain, which can then cause sleep quality to get worse, triggering more weight gain. You'll learn more about sleep in chapter 11.

The Environment and Hormones

While we know much about these hormones and their actions, scientists are still researching the way the environment impacts our hormones, from substances in plastics (like BPA) to flame retardants in fabrics, in furniture, curtains, and carpets.

Chemicals in the environment, known as endocrine disruptors, may affect the body's endocrine system. In the body, endocrine disruptors may mimic naturally occurring hormones. In response, the body may respond by over-producing or under-producing the mimicked hormones and others. Endocrine disruptors have been linked with developmental, reproductive, brain, immune, and other problems.

Low doses of endocrine-disrupting chemicals may be unsafe. The body's normal endocrine functioning involves slight changes in hormone levels, and we know even these small changes can cause significant developmental and biological effects.

Did you know that your perfume could be making you fat?

It's not just your perfume or cologne. It's every toxic product you are putting on your skin and hair, and every toxin you are inhaling on a daily basis. It's the shower you take every day with no filter. It's the chemicals you breathe in from car fumes during your outdoor jog.

Cytochrome P450 comprises 50 different enzymes, and while they are found in all tissues of the body, the highest concentration is within liver cells, and are essential during phase I of liver detoxification. As the primary site of drug metabolism, the liver functions to detoxify and facilitate excretion of xenobiotics (foreign drugs or chemicals) by enzymatically converting lipid-soluble compounds to more water-soluble compounds.

This process is very micronutrient dependent. Daily toxins deplete your micronutrients. If you are micronutrient deficient, then it's likely your detoxification pathways aren't working properly. This can result in toxins that accumulate in the body—such as that perfume you spray on yourself every day—which can interfere with fat burning. If your detoxification pathways are constantly being used to do the job of dealing with these toxins, they aren't available to do other fat burning jobs, such as creating brown adipose tissue, which is crucial for maintaining core body temperature and energy balance.

Chapter 3: The Food Groups

To survive, human beings need to consume several distinct types of organic and inorganic molecules. In addition to water, the nutrients you need are proteins, fats, carbohydrates, minerals, and vitamins. The big three—protein, fats, carbohydrates—are called macronutrients. Here's a review of each type, as well as a look at the "odd man out," alcohol.

Protein

Protein is a macronutrient essential in building muscle mass. It's commonly found in animal products, though is also present in other sources, such as nuts and legumes. Chemically, a protein molecule is made from a long chain of amino acids, each linked to its neighbor through a covalent peptide bond. Proteins are therefore also known as polypeptides.

Amino acids are organic compounds made of carbon, hydrogen, nitrogen, oxygen, or sulfur. Amino acids are the building blocks of proteins, and proteins are the building blocks of muscle mass.

It's important to understand that your body makes its own proteins from the available supply of amino acids. The protein in your body is genetically your own, just as the protein in your ribeye steak is genetically unique to that cow. Therefore, when your digestive system receives protein from any source, the protein itself is useless. It's genetically foreign. To be useful, it must be broken down into its component amino acids, which are ubiquitous. Like a bricklayer building a house from generic bricks, your body then uses these everyday amino acids to build your unique proteins.

Fats

All fatty acids have a similar chemical structure. Generally, they consist of a straight chain of an even number of carbon atoms, with hydrogen atoms along the length of the chain and also at one end of the chain. At the opposite end of the chain is a carboxyl group (—COOH). It is the carboxyl group that makes it an acid (carboxylic acid). Slight differences in structure translate into crucial differences in form and function. For example, if the carbon-to-carbon bonds are all single, the acid is said to be saturated. If any of the bonds are double or triple, the acid is unsaturated and is more reactive.

Fats are critical to many bodily functions. Triglycerides, cholesterol, and other essential fatty acids are not made by your body; you have to consume them. They store energy, insulate us, and protect our vital organs. They act as messengers, helping proteins do their jobs. They also start chemical reactions that help control growth, immune function, reproduction, and other aspects of basic metabolism.

Many foods naturally contain fats, including dairy, meats, poultry, seafood, eggs, seeds, nuts, avocados, and coconuts.

In the 1960s, dietary fat came under scrutiny from scientists because of the perceived behavior of different kinds of fats in the bloodstream. The idea was that certain fats helped to clog your arteries, leading to heart attacks and strokes. Initially, the clarion call was against all dietary fats. Hence began the "low-fat" food industry, which has become enormous, and which has generally replaced fats in processed foods with sugar and salt, leading to other health consequences.

Fats are highly complex and varied. There are four major types in the foods we eat:

1. Saturated fats

2. Trans fats

3. Monounsaturated fats

4. Polyunsaturated fats

The four types have different chemical structures and physical properties. The scientific establishment has grouped them into two types. These "experts" say saturated and trans fats are "bad" fats. They tend to be more solid at room temperature (like a stick of butter). They are primarily found in animal products like beef and pork, and in dairy foods like butter, margarine, cream, and cheese.

The so-called "good" fats are monounsaturated and polyunsaturated fats, which tend to be liquid (like liquid vegetable oil). You'll learn later in the book why some of these vegetable oils are the *worst* fats you can put inside your body.

Monounsaturated fats are found in avocados and peanut butter; seeds, such as pumpkin, sesame, and sunflower; and nuts, like almonds, hazelnuts, cashews, and pecans. They are also found in plant oils, such as safflower, sesame, canola, olive, and peanut oils.

Polyunsaturated fats include omega-3 fatty acids and omega-6 fatty acids. They are found in fish like salmon, mackerel, herring, tuna, and trout; in plant-based oils like soybean, corn, and safflower oils, and they're abundant in walnuts, flaxseeds, and sunflower seeds.

According to conventional wisdom, fats have different effects on the cholesterol levels in your body. The so-called bad fats— saturated fats and trans fats—supposedly raise the levels of bad cholesterol (LDL) in your blood. LDL cholesterol is said to form plaque in your arteries and increase your risk of cardiovascular disease and stroke.

But science is evolving. The nutritional axiom that saturated fat is bad for you continues to fall apart as a steady stream of new books and studies on this topic hit the media.

In the Keto Flex lifestyle, you should eat saturated fat. The benefits of saturated fat are innumerable: they taste delicious and help satisfy your appetite (which is very important if you're trying to lose weight), they help power your brain, help you optimize hormone levels, help you use fat for fuel (you become a fat burner instead of a sugar burner), and they will help you function optimally while burning fat at the same time.

As for trans fats, as the result of government regulation, they have been all but eliminated from foods in America.

The so-called good fats—monounsaturated fats and polyunsaturated fats—are said to lower the levels of bad cholesterol and are beneficial when consumed as part of a healthy dietary pattern. They raise the level of good cholesterol (HDL), which picks up excess LDL in the blood and moves it to the liver, where it is broken down and discarded.

Here's the bottom line: trans fats and vegetable oils (canola, corn, soybean, etc.) will raise your bad cholesterol. These bad guys stick to your arteries and cause heart disease, joint pain, inflammation, autoimmune diseases, and a host of other health problems. They are very unstable and akin to drinking liquid poison because they create destruction at the cellular level. Removing them from your diet as much as possible will result in a big drop in inflammation and a huge increase in energy levels. More on this important topic later in the book.

Carbohydrates

The third major macronutrient, carbs are the sugars, starches, and fibers found in many fruits, grains, vegetables, and milk products. They are called carbohydrates because, at the chemical level, the molecules contain carbon, hydrogen, and oxygen.

Like all macronutrients, your body cannot make carbs; it has to get them from the food you eat. They are classified as either simple or complex. The difference between the two forms is the chemical structure and how quickly the sugar is absorbed and digested.

Generally speaking, simple carbs contain just one or two sugars, such as galactose (found in milk products) and fructose (found in fruits). These single sugars are called *monosaccharides*. Carbs with two sugars, such as sucrose (table sugar), lactose (from dairy) and maltose (found in beer and some vegetables), are called *disaccharides*. They are digested and absorbed quicker and easier than complex carbs.

Complex carbs, called *polysaccharides,* have three or more sugars. They are often referred to as starchy foods and include beans, peas, lentils, peanuts, potatoes, corn, parsnips, whole-grain breads, and cereals.

In the digestive system, carbs are broken down into molecules of sugar, such as glucose and fructose. The small intestine absorbs these smaller units, which then enter the bloodstream and travel to the liver. The liver converts all of these sugars into glucose, which is carried through the bloodstream. Accompanied by insulin, which acts as a transporter, the glucose enters the cells, where it's converted into energy for basic body functioning and physical activity.

If the glucose is not immediately needed for energy, the body can store some of it in the liver and skeletal muscles in the form of glycogen, which as you recall are basically clumps of glucose molecules clumped around a small central core. Once those glycogen short-term stores are full, carbs are stored as fat.

Dietary fiber is a form of carbohydrate that resists digestion in the human gut. (In contrast, cows and other ruminants can digest plant fibers, such as hemicellulose and cellulose. This allows them to derive nourishment from forages and industrial byproducts that humans cannot digest).

There are two basic types of dietary fiber.

Soluble fiber dissolves in water to form a gel-like material. It's found in oats, citrus fruits, beans, apples, carrots, peas, barley, and psyllium.

Insoluble fiber resists digestion and promotes the movement of material through your digestive system. It's found in wheat bran, nuts, whole-wheat flour, potatoes, and beans, and in vegetables including cauliflower and green beans.

Micronutrients

In addition to water, protein, fat, and carbohydrates, to stay healthy your body needs various minerals and vitamins that it cannot make itself. Although only required in small amounts, micronutrient deficiencies can have devastating consequences.

Micronutrients can be divided into four categories: water soluble vitamins, fat soluble-vitamins, macrominerals, and microminerals (or trace minerals).

Water-soluble vitamins include ascorbic acid (vitamin C) and eight B-vitamins:

- Vitamin B1 (thiamine)

- Vitamin B2 (riboflavin)

- Vitamin B3 (niacin)

- Vitamin B5 (pantothenic acid)

- Vitamin B6 (pyridoxine)

- Vitamin B7 (biotin)

- Vitamin B9 (folate)

- Vitamin B12 (cobalamin)

Because they are not fat soluble, the body's tissues cannot hold them, and any excess is flushed away by the kidneys. Therefore, you need a steady supply. Overdosing is unlikely but taking a megadose of some water-soluble vitamins such as vitamin B6 can lead to potentially dangerous side effects.

Fat-soluble vitamins are vitamins A, D, E, and K. They are soluble in organic solvents and are absorbed and transported in a manner similar to that of fats. Your body can store them for a few days, and in some cases up to six months. Given that fat-soluble vitamins can accumulate in the body, mega dosing is likely to lead to toxicity.

Macrominerals are needed to perform specific roles in your body. They include calcium, phosphorus, magnesium, sodium, potassium, chloride, and sulfur. You must get them from foods you eat, or supplements. They are extremely important to good health. For example, a deficiency in magnesium, also known as hypomagnesemia, may result in twitches, tremors, muscle cramps, seizures or convulsions, mental disorders, osteoporosis, fatigue, high blood pressure, and asthma.

Microminerals are needed in very small amounts. They are iron, manganese, copper, iodine, zinc, cobalt, fluoride, and selenium. But just because you need a tiny amount does not lessen their importance. For example, iron is required to make hemoglobin, a protein in red blood cells that carries oxygen from the lungs to all parts of the body, and myoglobin, a protein that provides oxygen to muscles. Your body also needs iron to make some hormones. If you had insufficient iron in your diet or in supplements, you'd develop iron deficiency anemia. Its symptoms include extreme fatigue, chest pain, fast heartbeat, shortness of breath, headache, dizziness or lightheadedness, and other serious problems.

Alcohol

There's one more type of substance we consume—alcohol. It's in its own special category of food, if you can call it that. Ethanol —the stuff we drink—has 7 calories per gram, while protein and carbohydrates have 4 calories per gram and fat has 9 calories per gram. Beyond its calories, ethanol contains no nutrients such as fiber, protein, vitamins, or minerals. This is why many people refer to alcohol as a source of "empty" calories. And the body cannot store alcohol, so it metabolizes alcohol completely differently from the way it metabolizes carbohydrates, proteins, and fats.

Obviously, if you consume alcohol in beer or wine, you're getting a hefty dose of carbohydrates. And if you consume a cocktail like a tasty margarita, you can add sugar to the mix. Such concoctions are not good for a Ketogenic approach and must be avoided.

But how about a vodka on the rocks? No sugar, no carbs from grape or grain. Just ethanol and water. Pure calories.

In fact, back in 1964 a slender bestseller called *The Drinking Man's Diet*, by Robert Cameron, who for some peculiar reason wrote under the pseudonyms "Gardner Jameson and Elliott Williams," touted a low-carb diet as a way to have your steak and martini, too. If you cut out the sugar and carbs, and ate lots of protein, moderate alcohol intake was no problem. The subtitle of the book was, *How to Lose Weight with a Minimum of Willpower*. Wow! It sounded like a gift from heaven! Readers agreed, and it sold 2.4 million copies in 13 languages. But despite its Swingin' Sixties, Rat Pack appeal, the diet contained this nugget of truth: if you really limited yourself to 60 grams of carbohydrates per day, you could lose weight. A limit of 60 grams of carbohydrates (about three slices of bread) effectively removes most sugars and starches from your diet. The result will be calorie restriction and weight loss, even if you don't exercise.

Your Body's Fuel Priorities

Imagine you live in a remote cabin in the mountains. Winter is coming, and your only source of food is your pantry. With the air turning frosty, you need to stock up on provisions.

Let's say your food comes in five varieties or types. They are differentiated only by their "shelf life"—that is, how long you can preserve them. From time to time throughout the winter, you might get new supplies of each type—but you can't be certain of that.

Type 1 – Edible for one day; therefor does not belong in the pantry.

Type 2 – Edible for one week.

Type 3 – Edible for one month.

Type 4 – Can be stored in the pantry indefinitely.

Actually, this scenario is how our agrarian ancestors lived. They had to carefully budget their food.

Obviously, if you had a lick of sense, you'd eat the Type 1 food right away, no matter what it was. You'd save the other types for later. It would be insanity to eat the Type 4 food right away, wouldn't it?

When you ran out of Type 1 food, only then would you eat Type 2. When that was gone, you'd move on to Type 3.

You'd save your Type 4 food for as long as possible. By pursuing this strategy, you'd get the most from your food supply, and none would be wasted.

This is exactly what your body does; it first uses and digests the nutrients it cannot store. The nutrients it can store for later, it will. This is called your oxidative priority. Maria Emmerich explained this process brilliantly on The Keto Kamp Podcast.

This oxidative priority was systematized thousands of years ago, when food was scarce. In those days, it was certain that by the end of the winter, you'd be consuming Type 4 food—the edibles you had been storing in your pantry for months. Rarely would Type 4 food last from year to year. You *needed* it.

Times have changed! For billions of people in developed nations, food is plentiful. In fact, there's more than enough food to keep the pantry full, month after month, year after year. You can't pack food into your pantry fast enough. You never consume it. It just gets bigger and bigger.

Keto turns back the clock and allows your system to function the way it was designed thousands of years ago. By "shorting" you on the easy-to-burn fuels, it makes you utilize the fuel that you normally store away in your pantry—your fat cells. Here, the oxidative priority is alcohol (burned immediately), then carbs, then protein, and finally fats. In the typical SAD diet, the fats are stored for later use—but "later" never comes! In the Keto Flex lifestyle, these stored fats are called into action and used as fuel, which is what nature intended.

Chapter 4: Fasting—The Physician Within

When people think of fasting, the image that most often comes to mind is a skinny guy wearing a simple robe, sitting cross-legged in a monastery on a mountaintop. It has a decidedly spiritual context, in which the cleansing of the body is connected to the cleansing of the soul. In such a context, fasting is not connected to "real life," in which you have to go to work, get the kids off to school, clean the house, and do all the mundane stuff we do every day.

In the Keto Flex lifestyle, we look at fasting differently. Responsible, smart fasting is meant for everyday life. It plays an integral role in your daily health and well-being, and therefore you need to know as much as you can about it.

Fasting Vs. Starving

The first, and most important, distinction to make is between fasting and starving.

The difference is this:

Starving is what happens when, *against your will,* your access to food is restricted or shut off, causing your health to suffer, and perhaps even leading to death. Sadly, throughout human history, starvation has been a constant problem, even today.

Fasting is when, in an environment where food is readily available, you *choose* to restrict your food intake, in order to achieve a rational goal.

Under the overall umbrella of intentional food deprivation, there are two key sub-categories that need to be mentioned.

1. Hunger strikes. This is when you intentionally refuse food not because you want to improve your health but because you wish to draw attention to a political or social issue. In the United States, a large-scale hunger strike started on July 8, 2013 at Pelican Bay State Prison in California. The hunger strike was organized by inmates in long-term solitary confinement in the Security Housing Unit (SHU) in protest of inmates being housed in solitary confinement indefinitely simply for having ties to gangs. Over 29,000 inmates took part in the protest, which ended on September 5, 2013. At around the same time, another hunger strike at High Desert State Prison was to demand cleaner facilities, better food and better access to the library.

If sufficiently committed to their cause, human beings are capable of willfully starving themselves to death. In 1981, Irish republican prisoners held at Maze Prison, near Belfast, went on a hunger strike. When it was all over, ten prisoners had died. The first, IRA member Bobby Sands, started his strike on March 1, and after 66 days of not eating anything, he died on May 5. For the ten, the average period until death was between 60 and 70 days. The tenth striker, Michael Devine, died on August 20, after 60 days. In each case, the coroner recorded verdicts of "starvation, self-imposed."

Then we have the Guinness World Record for the longest recorded fast. His name was Angus Barbieri. This Scotsman went 382 days without food. His starting weight was 450 pounds, and his ending weight was 180 pounds. He was medically supervised, and doctors tracked his electrolytes and blood work throughout.

I would argue that while Angus didn't put food in his mouth for 382 days, he was "eating" from his body fat. He had a lot of fuel to consume!

2. Eating disorders. Particularly among adolescent girls, eating disorders present themselves as an unhealthy relationship to food, in which feeding oneself has become intertwined with a deeply rooted psychological problem. It may be difficult for observers to understand this, but to the person with an eating disorder, their extreme actions represent an *agreeable solution* to a more painful psychological problem, and bring very real emotional relief.

Anorexia nervosa is characterized by a distorted body image springing from an unfounded fear of being overweight. Patients literally see themselves as fat even when self-starvation has made them emaciated.

Binge eating disorder typically takes the form of eating unusually large amounts of food in relatively short periods of time and feeling a lack of control during binges.

Bulimia nervosa involves secret bingeing—eating large amounts of food with a loss of control over the eating—followed by purging in an effort to get rid of the unwanted calories in an unhealthy way. Methods of purging include forced vomiting, excessive use of laxatives or diuretics, and extreme or prolonged periods of exercising.

Pica is an eating disorder that involves eating things that are not considered food. People with pica crave and ingest non-food substances, such as ice, soap, pebbles, paper, dirt, hair, cloth, soil, chalk, laundry detergent, wool, or cornstarch.

Rumination disorder is a condition in which a person regurgitates food they have previously chewed and swallowed, re-chews it, and then either re-swallows it or spits it out. Rumination disorder can result in weight loss and severe malnutrition that can be fatal.

Orthorexia—not yet recognized as a separate eating disorder by the current *Diagnostic and Statistical Manual of Mental Disorders* (DSM)—manifests itself as an obsessive focus on healthy eating with no rational reason or goal. The affected person may eliminate entire food groups, leading to malnutrition, difficulty eating outside the home, severe weight loss, and emotional distress. Their self-worth, identity, or satisfaction is dependent upon how well they comply with their irrational, self-imposed diet rules.

All of these disorders require mental health counseling or psychiatric treatment, and can take years to resolve. Note that none of them involve setting a rational goal and then working to meet that goal; they are all about a morbid relationship with food stemming from a deep-seated emotional problem.

Ancient Fasting

Fasting—the deliberate and rational restriction of food intake to reach a stated goal—has a long and storied history.

The Bible makes frequent references to fasting. In the Old Testament, fasting fell into two categories: private and public. Private fasts were seen of acts of personal penance, while prayer, supplication, and sackcloth accompanied public fasts. When Moses ascended Mt. Sinai to receive the Ten Commandments, he fasted as an act of self-purification: "So he was there with the Lord forty days and forty nights. He neither ate bread nor drank water. And he wrote on the tablets the words of the covenant, the Ten Commandments." (Exodus 34:28)

And when John the Baptist lived in the desert, he subsisted on a very restricted diet: "Now John wore a garment of camel's hair and a leather belt around his waist, and his food was locusts and wild honey." (Matthew 3:4) But wait—he lived on locusts and wild honey? When you think about it, that's a nutritionally complete diet. Locusts are about 50 percent protein, 19 percent fat, 16 percent crude fiber, 5 percent carbs, and 10 percent water. They are a good source of iodine, phosphorus, iron, thiamine, riboflavin, niacin, and have traces of calcium, magnesium, and selenium.

Honey is mainly fructose (about 38 percent) and glucose (about 32 percent), with remaining sugars including maltose, sucrose, and other complex carbohydrates.

If John the Baptist ate mostly locusts with a bit of honey now and then as a treat, and if he had access to a daily multivitamin pill, he would have been very close to a healthy ketogenic diet!

In the Greek and Roman era we see fasting used not only as a method of spiritual cleansing but also as a way to combat disease. It's important to remember that ancient "physicians" (if you can call them that) had no way of knowing the inner workings of a living human being. They had knowledge of anatomy from cadavers, but many basic organ functions—particularly the heart and the brain—were unknown. The causes of infectious disease—viruses and bacteria—were unknown. All they had was careful observation of human behavior under various conditions.

In the 5th century BCE, Greek physician Hippocrates recommended abstinence from food or drink for patients who exhibited symptoms of certain illnesses. He and other natural philosophers recognized that patients in certain disease states naturally experienced a loss of appetite. Since fasting was thought to be an important natural part of the recovery process, administering food during such states was unnecessary and possibly even harmful because you were fueling the disease. Hippocrates wrote, "To eat when you are sick, is to feed your illness."

Around the same time, it was written that when the Buddha was traveling in the region of Kasi, near present-day Varanasi, India, he addressed a sangha of monks, saying: 'I, monks, do not eat a meal in the evening. Not eating a meal in the evening, I, monks, am aware of good health and of being without illness and of buoyancy and strength and living in comfort. Come, do you too, monks, not eat a meal in the evening. Not eating a meal in the evening, you too, monks, will be aware of good health and... living in comfort." Thus, was born the tradition of Buddhist monks avoiding food intake after noon.

Five centuries after Buddha and Hippocrates, Plutarch wrote, "Instead of using medicine, better fast today."

Fifteen hundred years later, Philip Paracelsus, the Swiss founder of the science of toxicology during the German Renaissance, wrote, "Fasting is the greatest remedy—the physician within."

And good ol' Benjamin Franklin, one of America's Founding Fathers and a man who knew a lot about a wide variety of topics, said, "The best of all medicines is resting and fasting."

Even today, we all know the common axiom, "Feed a cold, starve a fever."

Since self-imposed fasting involves exercising control of the physical body, many religions consider fasting a way to cultivate mental discipline, and use it in connection with prayer or meditation to heighten the spiritual experience and demonstrate adherence to custom. Fasting is particularly important for Christians during Lent, and Muslims during the holy month of Ramadan.

Yogic practices, including that of fasting, date back thousands of years. In the 20th century, Paramahansa Yogananda said, "Fasting is a natural method of healing."

In the Bahá'í faith, strict fasting—the complete abstention from both food and drink—is observed from sunrise to sunset during the Bahá'í month of 'Alá', from March 2 through March 20.

In Judaism, while Yom Kippur is the only fast day which is explicitly stated in the Torah, observant Jews fast six days of the year. On Yom Kippur, fasting as a means of repentance is mandatory for every Jewish man and boy above the bar mitzvah age and every Jewish woman and girl above the bat mitzvah age.

Therapeutic Fasting

In the United States, therapeutic fasting, intended to treat illness or maintain good health, became popular in the 19th century as part of the Natural Hygiene Movement. Much of the health and nutrition advice many people follow today—the role of fasting in the recovery of health, the advantages of a plant-based diet, the incredible healing powers of the body, and the importance of avoiding unnecessary drugs and surgery—were promoted by natural hygienists as far back as 150 years ago.

In 1928, Dr. Herbert Shelton (1895-1985) opened Dr. Shelton's Health school in San Antonio, Texas. He claimed to have helped 40,000 patients recover their health with a water fast. Nominated in 1956 by the American Vegetarian Party as candidate for President of the United States, he wrote, "Fasting must be recognized as a fundamental and radical process that is older than any other mode of caring for the sick organism, for it is employed on the plane of instinct."

In natural medicine, fasting is seen as a way of cleansing the body of toxins, removing diseased or dead tissues, and giving the digestive system a chance to reset to homeostasis. Such fasts typically allow only water, or sometimes clear fruit and vegetable juices. Fasting has also been used in the treatment of some kinds of cancer, autoimmune diseases, and allergies.

We usually think of food as giving us energy but digesting the food we eat actually *requires* energy. It is estimated that after a heavy meal, 65 percent of the body's energy must be directed to the digestive organs. During fasting, we rest our system from the constant onslaught of food. We re-direct our energy towards healing and recuperation. Our body can detox and repair cells and eliminate foreign toxins and natural metabolic wastes.

There's a misconception that foods give us energy, but it's the exact opposite. When we eat food, it takes massive amounts of energy to process that food. Earlier in the book, I referenced the University of Virginia study that showed a 14-hour time period for food to enter the small intestines. Chewing food and allowing the body to take macronutrients and assimilate them into micronutrients for distribution is a big task.

The analogy I like to give is one of a corporate employee named Sandra. Sandra works 9 a.m. to 5pm each day, putting in a full day of work. Imagine Sandra clocking out of her job after a long day of work and walking to her car. As she approaches her vehicle, thinking about going home to rest and recover, she receives a phone call from her boss asking her to come back to the office to work on an important project for the next 5 hours. Reluctantly, she goes back, and puts in the extra work. It is now 10 p.m., and Sandra is exhausted and ready to go home and rest. As she approaches her car again, she receives another phone call from her boss asking her to come back to the office to work on another project.

Imagine this happening to Sandra for days, and even weeks. She would begin to dysfunction. This is exactly what you're doing to your digestive system when we you're not practicing intermittent fasting.

From the perspective of the gut, you're not giving your gut the time it needs to rest in between meals.

After every meal, there is a little bit of postprandial (meaning the period after the meal) endotoxemia (meaning the presence of endotoxins in the blood). It can vary by the types of foods and fats that you're eating, but there always is a little bit of postprandial endotoxemia, and it can be worsened if you have leaky gut.

When you *don't* eat, you reduce that endotoxemia, so you're allowing and giving space for the body to be able to do its cleanup work to reduce inflammation and rebalance itself.

If you look historically at the number of meals that people ate 50 years ago compared to now, it used to be just three meals a day, and now its 5 or 6 meals per day. If this is the case with you, you're not giving your body that time to allow your blood sugar to drop, insulin levels to drop, and the internal balance to happen that improves your sensitivity to very important hormone, insulin.

When you're eating too many meals, you're not allowing that rest period that's necessary for the body to be able to hit the reset button in between. We were not meant to live with a continuous influx of calories!

One meal can create an energy expenditure from the body for up to 72 hours. That can take 70 to 80 percent of your energy levels. Think about that. I'm talking about the Standard American diet, which is indeed SAD.

Fasting Strengthens Intestinal Stem Cells

Stem cells are special human cells that are able to develop into many different cell types, ranging from brain cells to muscle cells. In some cases, they can also fix damaged tissues. You might say that stem cells are the body's ubiquitous, all-purpose cells from which all other cells with specialized functions are generated.

As you get older, your intestinal stem cells begin to lose their ability to regenerate. Because these stem cells are the source for all new intestinal cells, this decline can make it more difficult for an aging person to recover from gastrointestinal infections or other conditions that affect the intestine.

According to research from MIT biologists, this age-related loss of stem cell function could be reversed by a 24-hour fast. The researchers found that fasting dramatically improves stem cells' ability to regenerate, in both aged and young mice.

"Fasting has many effects in the intestine, which include boosting regeneration as well as potential uses in any type of ailment that impinges on the intestine, such as infections or cancers," said Omer Yilmaz, an MIT assistant professor of biology, a member of the Koch Institute for Integrative Cancer Research, and one of the senior authors of the study.

"This study provided evidence that fasting induces a metabolic switch in the intestinal stem cells, from utilizing carbohydrates to burning fat," added David Sabatini, an MIT professor of biology and member of the Whitehead Institute for Biomedical Research and the Koch Institute, and also a senior author of the paper. "Interestingly, switching these cells to fatty acid oxidation enhanced their function significantly." [11]

---

[11] MIT. https://news.mit.edu/2018/fasting-boosts-stem-cells-regenerative-capacity-0503#:~:text=The%20researchers%20found%20that%20fasting,both%20aged%20and%20young%20mice.&text=%E2%80%9CThis%20study%20provided%20evidence%20that,burning%20fat%2C%E2%80%9D%20Sabatini%20says

Reduced Risk of Breast Cancer

Researchers at the University of California, San Diego, reported that intermittent fasting reduced the risk of breast cancer in obese mice. They found that restricting eating to an eight-hour window, when activity was highest, decreased the risk of development, growth, and metastasis of breast cancer in mice.

The findings, published in the January 25, 2021 edition of *Nature Communications*, demonstrated how time-restricted feeding, which is a form of intermittent fasting aligned with the circadian rhythms of the subjects, improved metabolic health and tumor circadian rhythms in mice with obesity-driven postmenopausal breast cancer.

"Previous research has shown that obesity increases the risk of a variety of cancers by negatively affecting how the body reacts to insulin levels and changing circadian rhythms," said senior author Nicholas Webster, PhD, professor at UC San Diego School of Medicine. "We were able to increase insulin sensitivity, reduce hyperinsulinemia, restore circadian rhythms and reduce tumor growth by simply modifying when and for how long mice had access to food."

As we have seen before, elevated levels of insulin are damaging to the body. Research data indicated that elevated insulin levels in obese mice drove accelerated tumor growth. Artificially elevating insulin levels accelerated tumor growth, whereas reducing insulin levels could mimic the effect of the time-restricted feeding.[12]

Fasting for Brain Power

Our brain *function* doesn't decrease when we fast, but our brain *energy* does.

Here is some great research from my friend and author, health expert, and performance coach, Thomas DeLauer.

The "slowing down" of synaptic activity is the brain's way of conserving energy and giving itself a chance to recharge. This means the brain becomes more efficient. If you normally have 100 percent energy in your brain when you're not fasting, when you are eating a normal diet, it's going to be diversified throughout multiple areas of your brain. As far as synaptic energy goes and that whole synaptic process, let's say there are ten things to process. You have 100 percent, and 10 percent is given to 10 different areas of your brain. But when you're fasting, your body is becoming more efficient and it's turning off mechanisms that don't need to be used. So even if your overall energy directed in your brain is down to 50 percent instead of 100 percent, that 50 percent is being focused in one area at a time. This is why you can feel so

---

[12] ScienceDaily. https://www.sciencedaily.com/releases/ 2021/01/210125191806.htm

much more focused and so much more alert with the task at hand when you are fasting. We were hardwired this way when we were hunter-gatherers. You want to be focused and sharp to catch your next meal. I would rather have 50 percent less energy and have that energy focused on where I want it, then to have 100 percent energy and have that scattered all over the place in areas I don't really need.

When we are fasting, we are also not producing nearly as many neurotransmitters, things like serotonin, dopamine, and a bunch of others. While these neurotransmitters are important, they are metabolically costly to produce. They cost a lot of "internal money" for our body to make, meaning they are not exactly the best use of our body's energy. A lot of the time we produce more than we need. If we did the same thing we did with the synaptic activity and reduced the amount of neurotransmitters being produced, it would take a load off the central nervous system, and allow us to be more efficient and productive with how we use those neurotransmitters.

By reducing the release of neurotransmitters from synapses in the brain, fasting may also give the nervous system a break. It's also worth noting that high levels of synaptic activity (overactive synaptic activity) and high levels of neurotransmitter production are associated with neurodegenerative diseases including Alzheimer's, Huntington's, and Parkinson's.

Brain-Derived Neurotrophic Factor (BDNF)

Brain-derived Neurotrophic Factor, or BDNF, is like a brain fertilizer. It grows neurons and strengthens synaptic connectivity. When we are in a fasted state or high level of physical activity, we start producing more BDNF. It helps neurons grow and branch out towards each other, making it easier for neurons to communicate. This decreases the synaptic activity I mentioned earlier, which is very powerful. If we are *decreasing* the overall synaptic activity (the amount of communication going from neuron to neuron) but we are *increasing* the connectivity, we are increasing the potency of how that activity is communicated.

Put it this way: if you have two neurons that are communicating with each other, and you have a high amount of activity but a low-quality connection, you're basically trying to cram 10 percent of that energy across a broken bridge where things are falling off and the activity is falling through the cracks. When you are fasting, however, you have more neural connectivity with more efficient synaptic activity. Now with 50 percent of your energy going across a good, sturdy, unbroken and structured bridge, the communication will surely get from neuron to neuron.

BDNF not only grows neurons but it grows the bridges between them. BDNF also has antidepressant activity, which explains why when you are fasting and after exercise you feel pretty damn good. The combination of BDNF and the decreased activity within the brain ends up being very powerful. Lastly, BDNF grows this neural connectivity, and it grows it in the right areas of the brain. BDNF interacts with neurons in the hippocampus, cortex, and basal forebrain; all of these areas are involved in memory, focus, and overall sense of well-being. BDNF is a reason why you feel so damn good after a tough workout. It's why the music you listened to on your car ride *to* the gym sounds so much better on the car ride *from* the gym.

Intermittent fasting may also restore microbe diversity in the gut, increase tolerance against "bad" gut microbes, and restore the integrity of the intestinal epithelium.

Will the body go into starvation mode when you practice intermittent fasting? A recent study shows a 13 percent increase in the metabolism after 4 days of fasting.

How is this even possible? Allow me to explain.

It's okay not to stuff a muffin in your mouth every three hours.

The human body knows what to do.

Here's how it works:

When we go a period of time without food, incredible processes start in the human body.

There is no slowdown in metabolism. It's the complete opposite!

If you look at the study I posted, it shows a 13 percent increase in metabolism after fasting for four days.

How the heck is this possible?

When the body has gone a period of time without food, it starts to go into "survival mode," not "starvation mode." The body wants us to find our next meal so that we can stay alive.

What happens next is that it raises counter regulatory hormones. When we don't eat food, insulin levels drop, and we raise these counter regulatory hormones; they run counter to insulin.

Counter regulatory hormones include catecholamines, cortisol, glucagon, and growth hormone. This is our body's way of pumping us full of energy and focus so we can hunt for our next meal.

These counter regulatory hormones are why our metabolism increases with fasting! Adrenalin levels are increased so that we have plenty of energy to go get more food. For example, 48 hours of fasting produces a 3.6 percent increase in metabolic rate, not the so-called "metabolic shut-down." In response to a four-day fast, resting energy expenditure increased up to 14 percent. Rather than slowing the metabolism, instead the body accelerates it.[13]

Zombie Cells

Cells are like groceries: when they expire, they need to be thrown out – up to 70 billion every day.

We have cells within our body that begin to dysfunction, and they stick around causing us to age faster. Because they refuse to die, scientists call them senescent cells.

I call them *zombie cells*.

As they build up in your body, studies suggest they promote aging and the conditions that come with it, like osteoporosis and Alzheimer's disease.

Zombie cells start out normal but then encounter stress, like damage to their DNA or viral infection. At that point, a cell can choose to die or become a zombie, basically entering a state of suspended animation.

The problem is that zombie cells release chemicals that can harm nearby normal cells. That's where the trouble starts.

---

[13] TheFastingMethod.com. https://thefastingmethod.com/fasting-physiology-part-ii/

Researchers have also shown that transplanting zombie cells into young mice basically made them act older: their maximum walking speed slowed down and their muscle strength and endurance decreased. Tests showed the implanted cells converted other cells to zombie status.

One of the best ways to kill off these zombie cells is a process called *autophagy*.

Autophagy literally means, "eat thyself." It's the process of cleaning up damaged cells.

Think of the refrigerator you have in your kitchen. It has groceries, which all have an expiration date. What would happen if you let these groceries expire, and instead of throwing the expired food in the trash, you pushed them toward the back of the fridge?

You'd create a toxic environment! Mold, bacteria, and many other disgusting processes will occur.

The human body is like your refrigerator. It has cells, fats, and proteins, which all have expiration dates on them. If you aren't intentionally "taking out the trash" within your body, this toxic buildup can lead to diseases like cancer and Alzheimer's. Fasting helps your body get rid of these expired products! Fasting triggers the process of autophagy, which breaks down and recycles dysfunctional proteins, and cellular debris.

This is why world-renowned cancer doctor Thomas Seyfried said, "If you complete a seven-day water-only fast, once per year, you reduce your chances of getting any cancer by up to 95 percent!"

The opposite of autophagy is a pathway called mTOR, which is short for mechanic target of rapamycin. This pathway signals growth; it is anabolic. Think of bodybuilders, they get a ton of mTOR. This pathway can be healing in spurts, but can lead to problems if you are in a constant growth state. There's an art to balancing autophagy and mTOR, and this is the focus of my four pillars.

As we'll see in the pages ahead, when used as part of the Keto Flex lifestyle, intermittent, deliberate fasting can be an easy way (what's easier than *not* eating?) to clean out our reserves of glucose, burn ketones, lose weight, and feel great.

Chapter 5: The Case for Keto

If there's one word that strikes a combination of dread and cynicism in the hearts of overweight people, it's the word "diet." My goal with this chapter is to make the case for keto. A big shoutout to my friend Gary Taube's book on this subject. Keto is technically not a diet; it is a metabolic process. To most people who have tried to lose weight by dieting, the whole idea seems like an exercise in misery and failure.

Statistics support this impression.

A 2020 study in *The BMJ*, the weekly peer-reviewed medical trade journal published by the British Medical Association, examined the results of 121 random trials with nearly 22,000 patients enrolled in 14 diet plans. Each person followed a popular named diet and reported weight loss and changes in cardiovascular risk factors. The diets were macronutrient or "macro," which go beyond just calorie counting to tracking the macronutrients— grams of proteins, carbs and fats—you're eating within your calorie goal and ratios.

According to the study, evidence shows that over a period of six months, most macronutrient diets produced moderate weight loss and improvements in cardiovascular risk factors like blood pressure. Okay—so far, so good. The bad news is that after 12 months, the positive effect on weight reduction and improvements in cardiovascular risk factors largely vanished.

The study's authors also made the interesting observation that "differences between diets are, however, generally trivial to small, implying that people can choose the diet they prefer from among many of the available diets… without concern about the magnitude of benefits."[14]

A similar study from 2018, published in *Medical Clinics of North America*, followed 29 long-term weight loss studies, revealing that more than half of the weight lost by participants was regained within two years, and by five years, more than 80 percent of lost weight was regained.

Authors Kevin Hall, Ph.D., and Scott Kahan, M.D., noted, "Previous failed attempts at achieving durable weight loss may have contributed to the recent decrease in the percentage of people with obesity who are trying to lose weight, and many now believe that weight loss is a futile endeavor.[15]

When people first begin a weight-loss diet, they're usually very gung-ho, and it may be easy for them to make low-calorie meals or

---

[14] TheBMJ https://www.bmj.com/content/369/bmj.m696

[15] https://www.ncbi.nlm.nih.gov/pmc/articles/PMC5764193/

keep their refrigerator stocked with healthy food. But as the weeks and months drag on, their previous behavior starts to come back. They see their diet as punitive and start to "cheat." Or they think, "Great! I've lost weight. I should reward myself for enduring this torture."

To lose weight and enjoy good health, people need to make a total lifestyle change, not just follow a diet.

Restrictive dieting often means going against your body's stubborn instance to maintain your weight. This trait evolved in humans from long ago when food was scarcer and took more effort to acquire. By cutting out foods your body craves—particularly fats—you're fighting nature and setting yourself up for failure. If you're told not to eat things that you like, for the first few days you can resist eating them. But then your primal brain will start taking over and you'll want what you can't have.

The Triune Brain

While discussing the failure of diets, it's important to understand the decision-making structure of the brain.

In the 1960s, American neuroscientist Paul MacLean formulated the triune brain model, which postulated that the human brain had evolved into three distinct regions, forming a hierarchy. The three regions are as follows:

Reptilian or primal brain. This is the basal ganglia, a group of structures found deep within the cerebral hemispheres. It's responsible for the fight-or-flight survival response and other primal activities related to the survival of the organism.

Paleomammalian or emotional brain. This is the limbic system, a set of middle-layer structures in the brain that deal with emotions and memory. It regulates autonomic or endocrine function in response to emotional stimuli and is involved in reinforcing behavior.

Neomammalian or rational brain. This is the neocortex, a set of outer layers involved in higher-order brain functions including sensory perception, cognition, generation of motor commands, spatial reasoning, and language. This is the distinctly "human" part of the brain. Many other animals have robust primal and emotional brain functions.

While modern brain imaging technology has shown that MacLean's model is an oversimplification, it's very useful as an explanation for explaining how we humans can consciously think we should do something, and yet some inner control center in our own brain issues contradictory commands.

The typical scenario is easy to follow. Jane wanted to lose twenty pounds. She was forty years old and had been eating the same way her entire adult life. Little by little, the pounds kept appearing, and one day she decided enough was enough. She enrolled in a diet plan. Nutrisystem, Weight Watchers (inexplicably, now it's "WW"), Jenny Craig, Atkins—it doesn't matter which one she chose. This was a decision made by her rational brain. It said to her, "You have a weight problem, and the solution is to go on a diet. All you have to do is eat the food you're supposed to and not eat anything else, and the pounds will melt away." No problem, right? It's like choosing to drive your car at 55 MPH instead of 65 MPH because you know it will increase your gas mileage. Not a big deal, and you'll still get where you're going.

Jane went on her diet. It was unpleasant because she never really felt like she got enough to eat at mealtime. She felt deprived. Her stomach growled at her and she looked longingly at delicious food choices she couldn't have. But after a few weeks, she lost a few pounds. Her emotional brain was happy. She liked that her clothes fit better and she looked more slender. So far, so good.

But deep in her reptilian primal brain, alarm bells were ringing. Something terrible was happening! Jane's calories had been cut and the actual mass of her body was shrinking! For millions of years, the reptilian brain has been responsible for the most basic tasks of the survival of the species, and now it sensed a big threat. Whatever was happening out there in the "rational" world, it wasn't good. The weight loss conjured up primitive memories deep in her DNA of lean times and even starvation. That was unacceptable. It was time to put the brakes on this madness and *get some food*.

And so, by degrees, Jane started to cheat on her diet, as her reptilian brain cajoled her into eating more and restoring her body to the comfortable state it was in before she had begun her weight-loss program.

Sometimes, it's the emotional brain that pulls the plug on a diet. People eat for many reasons, not just to fill their bellies when they're hungry. Eating is bound up with all sorts of emotional baggage, and many people eat to relieve anxiety or depression. Emotional eating can suppress or soothe boredom, stress, sadness, anger, fear, and loneliness. Your emotions can become so intertwined with your eating habits that without thinking about what you're doing, whenever you're angry or stressed you automatically reach for a delicious treat. Eating sugary foods releases dopamine in your brain. The happy effect you feel when you eat a candy bar is real. When the reward system is activated, it reinforces the behavior that triggered it, making it more likely you'll carry out these actions again. Breaking these habits can be like kicking a drug habit.

The Keto Approach

If you accept the premise that it's the primal brain that overrides the rational brain's choice to go on a diet with restricted foods and calories, then it's easy to see how difficult it is to stay on a diet while the primal brain is fighting you every step of the way. You may *think* you want to lose weight, and you may even know you *must* lose weight, but it's like rolling a giant boulder uphill: The minute you relax, the boulder hurtles right back down to the base of the hill, where it wants to be. Then you feel guilty and ashamed, and vow never to do it again… until a few months later, when some new diet program is advertised on television.

Clearly, there are several problems with traditional weight-loss diets.

1. The food is unsatisfying. Following the beliefs established in the 1960s, many commercial weight-loss plans put you on a low-fat diet. They provide food that *looks* like the delicious treats you crave—even things like brownies and ice cream sundaes—but these pathetic low-fat imitations leave you feeling cheated.

Foods labeled fat-free, reduced fat, low-fat, or sugar-free don't equate with calorie-free, and they often contain additives like chemical fillers that make them decidedly unhealthy. In addition, reduced-fat foods have a perceived healthy image, and studies have shown that people tend to eat much more of these foods, either because they mistakenly believe it's okay to splurge on "low fat" foods or because the foods are so unsatisfying that they need to eat more. Therefore, when you see the terms "fat-free," "sugar-free," "low-fat," "skim milk," and "all-natural," think of the phrase "chemical shitstorm." Humans are the only species smart enough to create their own food, and dumb enough to eat it.

2. The food can be bad for your health. Many diet foods contain artificial sweeteners, which are universally worse for you than real sugar. When it comes to weight management, the microbiome is a huge key. Your microbiome consists of all the microbes—bacteria, fungi, protozoa, and viruses—that live on and inside your body. The microbiome may weigh as much as five pounds, with most of it in your digestive tract. Being zero calories, you would think artificial sweeteners would be beneficial for weight loss, but actually they are obesogenic, meaning they contribute to obesity. They do so by altering the microbiota composition of the gut. Under the influence of artificial sweeteners, gut bacteria changes to bacteria that is much more likely to cause fat storage and obesity.

Aspartame is the world's most widely used artificial sweetener. Marketed as NutraSweet, Equal, Sugar Twin, and AminoSweet, aspartame is present in more than 6,000 products, including Diet Coke and Diet Pepsi.

What is this stuff, exactly?

Aspartame is a synthetic chemical composed of the amino acids phenylalanine and aspartic acid, with a methyl ester. When consumed, your body breaks down the methyl ester into methanol, which may be converted into formaldehyde.

That's right—embalming fluid.

As U.S. Right to Know pointed out, the U.S. Food and Drug Administration first approved aspartame for some uses in 1981, saying it was "safe for the general population under certain conditions." But many scientists, then and now, have said the approval was based on suspect data and should be reconsidered.

Dozens of studies have linked aspartame to significant health risks including mood disorders, Alzheimer's disease, headaches and migraines, cancer, seizures, intestinal dysbiosis, cardiovascular disease, stroke, and dementia.

Evidence also links aspartame to increased appetite, weight gain, and obesity-related diseases. In fact, such evidence raises questions about the legality of marketing aspartame-containing products as "diet" drinks or weight loss products. In April 2015, U.S. Right to Know petitioned the Federal Trade Commission (FTC) and the Food and Drug Administration (FDA) to investigate the marketing and advertising practices of "diet" products that contain aspartame.[16]

3. "Grazing" ages you. Some popular diets advise you to eat five or six small meals throughout the day. The idea behind "grazing" is that it keeps you from getting too hungry and then overeating.

Just one of the many problems with grazing is that as you eat one snack after another, your body is constantly producing insulin. Insulin is your fat storage hormone, which signals your body to transport the extra glucose in your blood into your fat issues and prevent you from losing weight. Insulin is the neighborhood bully: when he comes around, all of your fat-burning hormones scatter. And each time you eat, you have an opportunity to overeat, even by a little bit. It's one more opportunity to make a bad choice.

Another problem is that your gut is designed to "re-set" after a meal, and a series of muscular contractions "sweeps" your small intestine from your stomach. This series of motions or contractions is called "peristalsis." Each time you eat, the sweeping motion starts again from the top. If you keep introducing food into the system, your small intestine never experiences a full wave of cleaning.

---

[16] USRTK.org. https://usrtk.org/sweeteners/aspartame_health_risks/

Although the large intestine has peristalsis of the type that the small intestine uses, general contractions called "mass movements" occur one to three times per day, propelling what is now feces toward the rectum. Mass movements are triggered by meals, as the presence of chyme (food being digested) in the stomach and duodenum prompts them. This is called the gastrocolic reflex, which controls the motility of the lower gastrointestinal tract following a meal in response to the stretch of the stomach with the ingestion of food. If you eat many small meals, your stomach never stretches, which will disrupt your gastrocolic reflex.

4. Dental health. While it's not a direct concern of this book, if you graze all day, you'll need to be committed to brushing your teeth after every snack. Really? Can you do that? I'll bet not. Having a coating of food on your teeth and gums all day is a ticket to cavities, gum disease, and bad breath. I've also seen upstream issues with the mouth factor into health results, including cavitations from tooth extractions, infected root canals, and mercury fillings. I highly recommend you listen to episodes 1 & 2 of The Keto Kamp Podcast to learn more. Seek out a biological dentist in your area to explore these issues. A great resource is IAOMT.org.

From Sugar Burner to Fat Burner

As we know, the body can burn only two types of fuel: there are fat burners and there are sugar burners. Regardless of the specific foods you choose to eat, the goal is to regularly enter into a state of ketosis, where your body is burning fat for fuel instead of sugar.

Most people who consume the Standard American Diet (SAD) are pure sugar burners. Their food intake produces a steady enlargement of fat cells, and this fat is never used for fuel. A sugar-burner is someone who is relying on glucose as the main source of fuel. When you are burning sugar, your brain is going to signal intense cravings for carbohydrate-rich foods. It's really not your fault; it's your default setting right now.

You may point out—and rightly so—that if you consumed nothing but the fat in your body as fuel, the end result would be starvation and death. This is exactly what happens to people during periods of extreme famine. Following total food deprivation, the effects of starvation (which we do not want) come in three stages:

1. Consumption of stored carbohydrates. Your body is capable of storing about 2,000 calories of carbohydrates: skeletal muscles store about 400 grams of glycogen, the liver stores 90 to 110 grams of glycogen, and your blood circulates roughly 25 grams as glucose. As you can imagine, in an active person, 2,000 calories lasts less than a day. Then it's depleted.

2. Ketosis. The body uses stored fat for energy. The breakdown occurs in the liver and turns fat into ketones. This phase, which is good, can last for weeks at a time. After fasting has gone on for one week, your brain will use these ketones and any leftover glucose. Using ketones lowers your need for glucose and your body slows down the breakdown of proteins.

3. Starvation. When the fat stores are too low, the body begins to turn to stored protein for energy. It begins to break down muscle tissues, which are full of protein. This is very bad. Protein is essential for our cells to work properly, and when it runs out, the cells can no longer function.

The cause of death due to starvation is usually an infection or other result of tissue breakdown, because the body is unable to gain enough energy to fight off bacteria and viruses.

The Keto Flex lifestyle does *not* recommend excessive fasting. As we'll see in the pages ahead, it calls for flexibility (hence "flex") and going back and forth between sugar burning and fat burning. You build up a little bit of fat, and then you burn it for fuel —just like putting food in your freezer and taking it out a week later. You don't just leave it there forever!

White and Brown Fat

Humans produce and store two primary types of fat cells—the familiar white adipose tissue (WAT) and brown adipose tissue (BAT), also called brown fat. There is also a third type, marrow adipose tissue (MAT), which is found in bone marrow, and whose function is the subject of research.

There is a big difference between WAT and BAT. White fat cells store energy in the form of a single large, oily droplet. They are otherwise relatively inert. In contrast, brown fat cells contain many smaller droplets, as well as chestnut-colored molecular machines known as mitochondria. These organelles can burn up the droplets to generate heat. Humans are mammals, and unlike reptiles, we generate our own internal heat. When the body is in a cold environment, these brown fat cells become activated, and through chemical reactions that use the oily droplets for fuel, literally generate heat. This helps us maintain our standard operating temperature, which for most people is 98.6 degrees Fahrenheit.

Babies have brown fat, presumably because they cannot yet shiver when cold, and so for warmth must rely more on burning brown fat. It was long assumed that brown fat disappeared in adults. It turns out that adults have brown fat, too. In 2009, three different groups independently published papers in the *New England Journal of Medicine* revealing their discoveries of active brown fat cells in healthy adults. Scientists have since been trying to figure out how to study brown fat more easily and in greater detail.

Experts believe that brown fat has many more benefits mostly due to its ability to burn more energy (calories) to be used for body heat. During this process, your body's internal temperature increases and helps reduce other fat deposits made of white fat, the type many of us need to have less of. Certain studies have even shown that brown fat can burn up to five times more calories than other types of body fat!

Interestingly, because cold conditions activate brown fat, our ancestors—even those a few generations back—may have benefitted from BAT's fat-burning capability because they lacked central heat. Occasionally being in a cold environment is good for you, but with today's climate-controlled, hermetically sealed buildings and cars, we don't experience changes in temperature the way our ancestors did. Studies have shown that people exposed to cold indoor temperatures—not super cold, just a brisk 63 degrees Fahrenheit—burn more calories from fat than people in a warmer environment.

The Rational Way to Eat

If you look at all the evidence, including how we have eaten over thousands of years and how our digestive system is designed, you have to conclude that for optimum efficiency and good health, intermittent fasting combined with a diet high in natural fats and protein and, low in carbohydrates is the way to go. The body is quite accustomed to using ketones as fuel, and it's been doing that for millions of years.

Of course, many people have questions about intermittent fasting, mostly fueled by all the myths about it—that if you fast, your body will cannibalize your muscles, or that your brain will shut down, or you'll feel so starved that the minute your fast ends, you'll gorge on too much food. These stories are all nonsense, and if you try intermittent fasting, you'll quickly find out for yourself. In the chapters ahead, we'll dive deeper in these myths and debunk them.

Chapter 6: Getting Started

While learning about problems and their solutions is good, what you want are *results*, and to get results, you need to take *action*.

We're talking about two questions: *what* you eat and *when* you eat it. Both are equally important. In the Keto Flex lifestyle, you can't pay attention to one without paying attention to the other. They go hand in hand.

Let's start with how the foods you eat can be used for energy.

Ketosis

The goal of the Keto Flex lifestyle is to ensure your body regularly enters into a state of ketosis.

What does that mean?

Ketosis is a metabolic state in which the blood contains a high concentration of ketones. These ketones are then used by the cells in the body for energy.

How does that happen?

When you sharply cut your intake of carbohydrates, you will experience lowered levels of circulating blood sugar (glucose) derived from those carbohydrates. In response, your body will look for energy elsewhere. It will start breaking down stored fat and changing it into molecules called ketone bodies. The process is called ketosis. Once you have ketones circulating in your blood, your cells will consume these ketone bodies to generate energy until you start eating carbohydrates again. Ketones can cross the blood-brain barrier and be used by the brain for fuel.

Our hunter-gatherer ancestors, who endured long periods of quasi-starvation as they searched for game, burned their body fat, resulting in entering ketosis and using ketones to fuel their brains.

How quickly does this happen?

Scientists say the shift from using circulating glucose to breaking down stored fat as a source of energy usually begins over two to four days of eating fewer than 20 to 50 grams of carbohydrates per day. Everyone is different, and the process is highly individualized. Some people need a more restricted diet to start producing enough ketones.

Why is this good?

It's good for many reasons, but primarily because instead of relentlessly storing fat, your body can reclaim it and use it for energy, which is precisely why it's there in the first place. Your body designed its fat cells to serve as a backup energy supply, and ketosis takes advantage of the thousands of "free" calories locked in your cells in the form of fat. We say "free" because they cost you nothing. You paid for them long ago, in the form of the food you ate weeks, months, or even years ago. Ketosis removes this excess fat and puts it to good use.

A good metaphor is in your home: your refrigerator and your freezer.

Your refrigerator is your short-term storage unit for food. Nothing stays in there very long. It contains the food you eat every day.

But let's say you have an excess of food. What should you do with it? Well, over many millions of years, your body has been trained to be thrifty. It believes that since a food shortage could happen at any time—and painful experience has proved this to be true over and over again—you need a backup supply of energy. If you got excess calories from a rice harvest or from killing a big woolly mammoth, then you needed to store them away for tomorrow. Your body does this in the form of fat. At home, you do this with a freezer. You store excess food in your freezer until you need to eat it.

But what happens if you never eat it, because your refrigerator is always full of fresh food? Then your freezer fills up. And because you're relentlessly thrifty, you buy another freezer. When that one is full, you buy another one. Eventually, you live in a house full of freezers, all full of food. The electricity bill is very high!

If one day you emptied out your refrigerator and there was no food in it, what would you do?

You'd go to the freezer and use some of your stored food. If you kept doing this, a little bit at a time, eventually you could get rid of some of your freezers.

Sadly, the "buy more freezers" scenario has been playing out in Okinawa, the island group in Japan that for centuries was known for the longevity and good health of its people.

During the postwar era up until the year 2000, Okinawa had the longest life expectancy in all prefectures of Japan and one of the longest in the world. The local diet consisted of green and yellow vegetables, fish, relatively smaller amounts of rice compared to mainland Japan, as well as pork, soy, and other legumes. The staple of the Okinawa diet was the Satsuma sweet potato, which unlike other carbohydrates does not have a large effect on blood sugar. The traditional Okinawan diet had only 30 percent of the sugar and 15 percent of the grains of the average Japanese dietary intake, which itself was better than the aptly named Standard American Diet, or SAD.

The traditional Okinawan diet brought many benefits including minimal weight gain with age, low body mass index (BMI) throughout life, and low risk from age related diseases. The diet was also rich in ingredients that were said to possess anti-aging and antioxidant properties, such as turmeric. Like many cultures, people in Okinawa believed in the healing power of food, which they regarded as medicine, and the reason to their longevity.

The postwar era changed everything. Okinawa was occupied by the U.S. troops for 27 years, from the end of World War II to May 1972, and the American presence still looms large in the form of fast-food chains. In 1948, Blue Seal ice cream arrived, and the U.S. company built a factory at Tengan military base to provide dairy products to the troops. The local population grew to love them. In 1963, American fast-food chain A&W introduced root beer, hamburgers, and curly fries to Okinawa. Now the island is crammed with franchise outlets of McDonald's, Burger King, KFC, Mos Burger, King Tacos, Subway, Mister Donut, and other purveyors of salt, sugar, and carbohydrates disguised as food. Not surprisingly, the life expectancy of young Okinawans, who never knew the local diet, has plummeted. Their digestive systems are taking in too many calories and storing the excess as fat, and the health problems are following right behind. Today, the legendary lifespan of Okinawans is a thing of history, and the residents are dying from Western diseases—heart attacks and diabetes—at the same rate as Americans.

The point is this: eat a healthy diet. Keep your refrigerator half full, and when it gets empty, leverage the power of ketosis by going to the freezer, taking some of that free food energy and enjoying it!

A Long History of Safety

Let's clear up one bit of misinformation about Keto, which is its safety. The first thing we need to make clear is that every person is an individual, and you should do your own research about any diet or nutritional plan that features certain foods over others. When in doubt, be sure to consult your physician. If this or any other diet plan has negative side effects, stop it and talk to your doctor.

The fact is keto is not a diet; it's a metabolic process. It is nothing new. Its origins are deep in human history as every single one of our ancestors did keto.

In ancient times, epilepsy and its scary seizures confounded natural philosophers, who attributed the disease to supernatural attacks from evil spirits.

The legendary Greek physician Hippocrates discovered that somehow—he did not know why—fasting was an effective therapy for combating epilepsy. As the centuries unfolded after Hippocrates, other physicians achieved the same results. They saw that the number and severity of epileptic seizures decreased if the patient fasted. There was a problem, though: prolonged fasting is not a long-term solution to anything, because the final outcome is death by starvation, which no one wants.

In 1911, worldwide interest in fasting as a means to treat epilepsy was revived when two Paris doctors known to us as Guelpa & Marie published a paper in which they described how they could *mimic* the effects of fasting by using a special high-fat, low-carbohydrate diet. With their diet, which their patients could stay on indefinitely, they helped 20 people control their epilepsy, and they recorded the entire process in a report.

In 1921, Dr. Russell Wilder, a pioneering researcher in diabetes and nutrition at the Mayo Clinic, developed Ketogenic Therapy, known as the classic Ketogenic Diet, for the treatment of epilepsy. Like Guelpa & Marie, he realized that you could mimic the positive effects of fasting over many months and even years with a special high-fat, low-carb, low-protein diet. The diet proved to be both perfectly healthy and effective against epilepsy. It was far more effective than phenobarbital and bromides, then the only available anticonvulsant medications. The ketogenic diet earned its place in the medical world as a therapy for pediatric epilepsy, and was widely used until its popularity waned with the introduction of antiepileptic agents such as phenytoin (Dilantin).

In 1994, interest in the Keto diet was revived when a little boy named Charlie Abrahams developed severe epilepsy that was unresponsive to medications, which gave him terrible side effects. After learning about the Keto diet in a medical textbook, his parents took him to Johns Hopkins Hospital in Baltimore, MD. Charlie began the diet, and within days his seizures stopped. He remained on the diet for five years. At last report, he lives on his own and remains seizure-free.

The family shared their story with the media, and thousands of letters poured in. Charlie's father, Jim Abrahams, was instrumental in bringing to the public the 1994 *Dateline* TV news magazine program, "An Introduction to the Ketogenic Diet," featuring his friend, actress Meryl Streep. The same year he created the Charlie Foundation to Help Cure Pediatric Epilepsy. In 1997 he wrote, directed, and produced *First Do No Harm*, a television movie starring Meryl Streep that was based on the true story of another child who also became seizure-free thanks to a Ketogenic diet. This fostered increased worldwide interest and spurred further research that has proven the effectiveness of the diet as a treatment for epilepsy.

In many studies, the ketogenic diet has been shown to be particularly helpful for conditions including infantile spasms, Rett syndrome, tuberous sclerosis complex, Dravet syndrome, Doose syndrome, and GLUT-1 deficiency.

Today, an epileptic seizure is defined as a transient symptom of abnormal excessive or synchronous firing of some or many of the brain's cells, or neurons. Why does fasting help control epilepsy? Science doesn't have the answer. It's like aspirin: no one knows precisely how it works, but it does work. In another twist to the story, while both intermittent fasting and the Ketogenic diet reduce epileptic episodes in children, scientists believe they are not identical treatments, and that they are effective through two different mechanisms.

A 2010 study suggested that episodic fasting, in addition to the diet, was even more effective than the diet alone in controlling seizures.[17]

The "Keto Flu"

As your body adjusts to any change of diet—especially one that is moving you towards better health—there may be some initial side effects. The most common and relatively minor short-term side effects of beginning the Keto Flex lifestyle may include nausea, vomiting, headache, fatigue, dizziness, insomnia, difficulty in exercise tolerance, and constipation. These symptoms are usually referred to as "keto flu," which is more accurately

---

[17] https://www.dana.org/article/epilepsys-big-fat-answer/

described as carbohydrate withdrawal symptoms. They usually resolve in a few days to few weeks.

Not all people will exhibit keto flu symptoms when going through the diet transition period. Some are able to switch to a keto diet with little-to-no side effects.

What causes the keto flu?

It's really very simple.

Carbohydrates are stored in the body with water. When you lower your carb intake, your body initially responds by excreting more water and retaining less. As you lose water, this may give you a quick "lean" look. Less carbs means less insulin release, causing the kidneys to release more sodium. This loss of sodium impacts the balance of other key electrolytes, including sodium, potassium, and magnesium. These are minerals that carry an electrical charge. Vital for health and survival, they spark cell function throughout the body, support hydration, and help the body produce energy.

As carb intake decreases and electrolytes are increasingly excreted from the body in urine, imbalances of these electrolytes trigger the keto flu symptoms.[18]

_____

[18] HVMN.com. https://hvmn.com/blogs/blog/ketosis-keto-electrolytes-tips-and-concerns

Ensuring adequate fluid and electrolyte intake can help counter some of these symptoms. Long-term adverse effects may include hepatic steatosis, hypoproteinemia, kidney stones, and vitamin and mineral deficiencies.[19]

The bottom line is that in clinical settings, the ketogenic diet has been used by doctors for nearly a century and is considered to be extremely safe.

The Classic Keto Diet and Its Variations

The typical "classic" ketogenic diet is called the "long-chain triglyceride diet." Triglycerides are a type of fat (lipid) commonly found in your blood. When you eat, your body converts any excess calories into triglycerides. These triglycerides are stored in your fat cells. The chain lengths of the fatty acids in naturally occurring triglycerides vary, but most contain 16, 18, or 20 carbon atoms.

Medium-chain triglycerides (MCTs) are triglycerides with two or three fatty acids having an aliphatic tail of 6 to 12 carbon atoms.

Long-chain triglycerides (LCT), which have fatty acids of greater than 12 carbons, behave differently from MCTs in that they

---

[19] Ketogenic diet. https://www.ncbi.nlm.nih.gov/books/NBK499830/#:~:text=A%20ketogenic%20diet%20primarily%20consists,5%25%20to%2010%25%20carbohydrates.

are absorbed directly into the portal circulation and transported to the liver for rapid oxidation.

In a clinical setting—when treating epilepsy—the typical long-chain triglyceride diet provides 3 to 4 grams of fat for every one gram of carbohydrate and one of protein. This high fat, low-carbohydrate diet has been in clinical use since 1921, and is provided by a neurologist working together with a registered dietitian.

When treating epilepsy, the ketogenic diet is not simply a short-term fix. As the Carson Harris Foundation noted, a patient typically stays on the diet with their seizures well controlled for two years. If the patient is taken off the diet, it's done gradually, over a period of several months or even longer. Just as can happen if seizure medicines are stopped suddenly, if the ketogenic diet is stopped all at once, the seizures may become much worse. In many situations, because the diet has led to significant seizure control, families sometimes choose to remain on the ketogenic diet for many years.[20]

Macronutrient Ratios

There are five types of ketogenic diets, distinguished by their macronutrient ratio by weight.

---

[20] https://www.carsonharrisfoundation.org/ ketogenic_diet_long_chain_triglyceride_diet_ketogenic_diet.php

All of them are a variation of classic Keto developed by Dr. Wilder, which is the strictest in its ratio of fat to protein and carbs, also called the macronutrient ratio. Classic Keto specifies a 4:1 ratio by weight, which means that there are four parts fat for every one part protein and one part carb. This is why, in a strict Keto diet, all food is weighed. Since fat has a higher caloric content versus protein and carb (fat has 9 calories per gram, while both protein and carb have just 4 calories per gram), in a classic Ketogenic Diet, 90 percent of calories come from fat, 6 percent from protein, and 4 percent from carbs.

Here's a table of the common variations of the classic Keto diet.

Macronutrient ratio by weight	Fat	Protein	Carb
Classic Keto (4:1)	90%	6%	4%
Modified Keto (3:1)	87%	10%	3%
Modified Keto (2:1)	82%	12%	6%
Modified Keto (1:1)	70%	15%	15%
Medium chain triglycerides (MCT) / Long chain triglycerides (1.9:1)	50% / 21%	19%	10%
Low glycemic index treatment (LGIT) (2:3)	60%	28%	12%
Modified Atkins (0.8:1)	65%	29-32 %	3-6%

As you can see, there's a wide range from which to choose, and you should find the one that works best for you.

While there are many variations of the keto diet, let's start with the classic keto diet that started it all.

Looking at the table, we can see the ratio, by weight, of fats to protein and carbs is 4:1:1. By weight, to consume 2,500 calories per day, your daily consumption would be fat = 250 grams (9 calories per gram), protein = 37.5 grams (4 calories per gram), and carbs = 25 grams (4 calories per gram). Your total daily food intake would be 312.5 grams.

By calories, its 90 percent fats, 6 percent protein, and 4 percent carbs. So if you were a man and you were aiming for 2,500 calories per day, then you'd need about 2,250 calories from fat, 150 calories from protein, and 100 calories from carbs.

What might that equal in real life?

Figuring out what to eat can get complicated because of two things.

1. Every human body is unique, and you may have your own diet goals. The amount of calories you will need to lose weight will depend upon your height and weight, your body mass index, your level of physical activity, age, and gender. Some people will lose

weight on 2,800 calories per day, while others need to get down to 2,000 calories per day.

2. Foods are chemically complex. Most foods contain some fat, some carbs, and some protein, in varying proportions. While a food may be high in fat, it may also add to the other columns as well. It can get tricky to make them add up to a specific number.

The modified keto diets exist because you are an individual, with your own needs and tolerances. You are the best judge of how you want to improve your health. As you'll see in the coming chapters, I have seen that increasing protein and lowering dietary fat produce incredible results. Keep in mind that your body can get its fat calories either from dietary fat or from your butt, hips, and thighs. You choose!

That's why the best solution is for you to just give it a shot and see how it works for you. There are foods that are generally "keto-friendly," and those that are "keto-unfriendly." The goal is to eat more keto-friendly foods, and as you get used to them, you can become more focused. I've seen over and over again how people say to themselves, "I could never eat a cheeseburger without a bun!" but once they try it a few times, they become accustomed to it, and soon the idea of eating a cheeseburger with a big dose of carbohydrates seems repellent. It takes time to wean yourself away from the foods that may provide short-term pleasure but in the long run make you feel gross. I teach my Keto Kamp Academy students how to develop a strong relationship with their body. There are mechanisms and receptors inside your body that give you signals when something is working and when something is not. Small tweaks lead to giant peaks. You aren't competing against anyone else doing the Keto Flex lifestyle; your only competition is with yourself. Our motto at Keto Kamp is to beat yesterday.

Ease into the Keto Flex Lifestyle

Any diet that shocks your system is not going to work. Recall the power of your reptilian or primal brain located in the basal ganglia. Not to mix too many animal metaphors, but this is the watchdog of your brain. It's always ready to detect the slightest threat to your safety and survival. Threats include any drop in the amount of food you normally consume during the day. So, if you suddenly go on a "crash diet," your primal watchdog will be alerted. You may be able to pat him on the head and placate him for a while, but eventually he'll start barking and creating a disturbance that you cannot ignore. He'll make you so uncomfortable and miserable that to shut him up, you'll run to the kitchen or to McDonald's and pound down a few thousand calories.

A common challenge is when you make a self-imposed deadline for dropping a certain number of pounds. You see your high school reunion approaching, or a summer vacation that will require bathing suits, and you think, "OMG! I've got to lose ten pounds in two weeks!"

Then you sign up for a fad diet or take weight-loss pills that promise to "melt away" your body fat. You hear testimonials from celebrities who had lost weight quickly this way, probably because they were paid to do it. It's easy to believe you can slim down for the long term by using a fad diet, supplements, or pills. But these strategies are unsustainable. You cannot take pills forever. You cannot walk around all day feeling hungry and deprived because you're eating crappy "low-fat, low-calorie" food. That vigilant watchdog in your primal brain is barking his head off and driving you crazy. It's only a matter of time before you go back—with a vengeance—to your customary eating habits.

In the following four chapters, I'll show you how you can ease yourself into the Keto Flex lifestyle, one Pillar at a time. Each Pillar is painless, and you should only take the next Pillar when you're comfortable. It will take time. Look at it this way. Unless you've been overweight since childhood, you've probably gained weight as an adult. The Centers for Disease Control and Prevention (CDC) reports that the average person typically puts on one to two pounds per year from early adulthood through middle age. The

CDC's numbers show the average man in his twenties weighs around 185 pounds. But by his thirties, he's closer to 200 pounds. The average woman's weight goes from about 162 to 170 pounds over the same period. So, let's say that like many Americans, you've gained 20 pounds over a period of ten or fifteen years. Why do you think it would be possible to drop those 20 pounds in even one year? That would require a massive effort, and that watchdog in your primal brain would be barking in your ear every step of the way. The odds of your giving up and putting the weight right back on again are very high.

You've heard the term "yo-yo dieting." It's a very real phenomenon. On a daily basis, millions of Americans are looking for a new diet to try. According to the CDC, almost half of U.S. adults are on a diet at any given time. Women are more concerned with weight loss than men (56.3 percent and 42.2 percent, respectively), and what is truly astonishing is that according to various sources, the average dieter tries between 55 to 130 diets in their lifetime.

A 2020 survey conducted by Love Fresh Berries, a U.K. fresh fruit trade organization, found that people don't stick to these fad diets for very long. They usually abandon them after an average of just six days. Over half of respondents (52 percent) reported they were "really confused" about which of these fad diets were intended for a short-term period, and which were sustainable over long periods of time.

The survey revealed that when it came to fad dieting, a lack of understanding and readily available information was a major obstacle. Overall, more than half were "baffled" regarding which foods should and shouldn't be cut out of their eating habits, and 20 percent of respondents said that they had no idea where to go for reliable dietary information.[21]

The Keto Flex diet—or lifestyle, to be more accurate—is designed to be your roadmap to good nutrition for the rest of your life (barring, of course, the occasional slip). I always say, "It's never about the set-back, it's about the get-back. The Keto Flex lifestyle is not carved in stone. It's a road map, not a set of commandments. It's not punitive. It's not designed to make you suffer. To the contrary, it should make you feel really good!

The plan unfolds in four Pillars, which you take in easy succession.

1. Adapt. Your body learns to switch from using sugar as its sole fuel source to occasionally using fat.

2. Fast. After you become keto adapted, you can move up to implement intermittent fasting, so you can burn body fat and heal

---

[21] https://www.studyfinds.org/food-fads-the-average-adult-will-try-126-different-diets-during-their-life/

yourself. During this pillar, we practice various intermittent fasting strategies as we build up your fasting muscle.

3. Phase. This is where you are going to help your cells use fat as its only fuel source for a designated period of time. We practice the carnivore diet and phase out all carbohydrates for 30 days.

4. Flex. This is where you develop the flexibility to intentionally go in and out of ketosis. The most common challenge with an ordinary keto diet is inherent to the diet. Many people who do a keto diet can't stick to it, or they have cravings, or they find the longer they stick with it, the more challenging it is to keep the weight off. As you'll discover, this flex approach is the differentiator. What I will show you in Pillar 4 is that a long-term keto diet can actually cause weight gain and hormone imbalance, and how my Keto Flex approach prevents this and keeps you on the path to your ideal weight and perfect health.

Chapter 7: Pillar 1—Adapt

Your entry into the Keto Flex lifestyle has been carefully designed to be pleasant. It will not arouse the ire of the vigilant watchdog in your primal brain. We respect the watchdog and know his power. Therefore, every effort will be made to keep him peacefully sleeping.

The program has been designed to be built on four Pillars. You can take these four Pillars at your own pace.

Let's begin the process of becoming fat (keto) adapted.

What does this mean?

First, let's review how your body processes food into energy.

When you eat food—a mix of carbs, protein, and fat—your digestive system converts molecules from the carbs and proteins into molecules of glucose, which are transferred into your bloodstream and raise your blood sugar level.

As blood glucose levels rise, the pancreas secretes insulin. This hormone performs several key functions. It acts as a transporter, carrying glucose to the cells in the body where it's to be used as an energy source.

As a side note, in type 2 diabetes, which is at near-epidemic levels in the industrialized world, the muscle, fat, and liver cells build *insulin resistance*. They don't allow insulin to carry the glucose into the cell, which is bad because every cell must have glucose to survive. I know, it sounds weird that your cells would refuse to accept a delivery of groceries, but that's what happens. In response, the pancreas churns out more insulin. For a while, this strategy works, and your blood sugar levels stay normal. But over time, your pancreas isn't able to keep up, and your blood sugar levels rise until you have prediabetes.

Back to our story. Blood glucose enters liver cells, called hepatocytes, where the insulin stimulates the action of several enzymes, including glycogen synthase (the conversion of glucose into glycogen). While both insulin and glucose remain plentiful, glucose molecules are added to the clumps of glycogen.

Additionally, when there is excess glucose in the bloodstream, known as hyperglycemia, insulin encourages the storage of glucose as glycogen in the liver, muscle, and fat cells. These stores can then be used at a later date when energy requirements are higher or when food is scarce, such as when you're fasting. As a result of this, there is less insulin in the bloodstream, and normal blood glucose levels are restored.

In simplified form, the "glucose chain" goes like this: you eat food, releasing glucose into the bloodstream. The glucose travels to the liver, where it's combined with insulin to make glycogen, which can be stored.

Think of glycogen as your sugar reserves. I'm going to compare these sugar reserves to the refrigerator in your kitchen. It's easy access—you just open the door and pull out fresh food, ready to eat.

Your fat stores are more difficult to get to. Think of your fat stores as the freezer in your basement (if you're a hunter, you know exactly what I'm talking about). The food in your freezer is more difficult to access—you have to go downstairs, get the frozen food, and then thaw it out.

Your glycogen stores (refrigerator) can store about 2,000 calories. It has limited capacity. Anything more is stored as fat (the basement freezer) has almost unlimited reserves. Plus, you can always install more freezers—that is, add fat cells to your expanding waistline.

Recall we talked about being a "fat burner" vs a "sugar burner." Here's a handy equation to remember:

High insulin levels = Sugar burner

Low insulin levels = Fat burner

What's fascinating is that fat is the only type of food that has almost no effect on insulin. You can eat all the fat you want and it will not give you the insulin spikes that carbs do.

This is why the first Pillar in the Keto Flex lifestyle is to remove most of the carbohydrates in your diet and replace them with healthy fats and protein.

"Easy for you to say," I can hear from my dear readers.

Actually, it is pretty easy. That's because you don't have to count calories, or weigh your food, or do anything like that. You start by eating three times a day until you feel full, and you don't eat between meals. But because you're truly full at mealtime, you'll be amazed at how easy it is to skip eating snacks between meals. You won't feel hungry until it's time for your next meal.

"How is that possible?" you ask.

Because crappy, low-fat "diet" meals do not satisfy you! You eat the prescribed meal, and you still feel hungry, and as the hours pass your hunger only grows. By mid-morning, mid-afternoon, or midnight, you're *desperate* for something to eat. To solve the problem, you'll probably reach for a candy bar or, even worse, one of those sugary, 500-calorie specialty coffee drinks. Such "carbo bombs' only serve to accelerate your hunger and make you even more miserable. It's a vicious downward spiral.

In reality, dietary fat tastes good, satisfies your hunger, and makes you feel comfortably full. As NBC News reported, studies have found that healthy unsaturated fats (like monounsaturated or polyunsaturated omega-3 or omega-6 fats) have a positive effect on satiety and help to regulate your appetite by controlling the release of appetite hormones.

Adding enough fat and protein to your meal helps slow down the rate at which your stomach empties during digestion; and the longer some food remains in your stomach, the longer the sense of fullness lasts—sending that signal of satiation to your brain.[22]

This keeps the watchdog in your primal brain happy and relaxed!

As an added bonus, because fats taste good and are satisfying, they allow you to reduce the amount of sauces and sugar added when you cook. Fat boosts flavor, and enhances the taste of both sweet and salty foods.

Let's talk more specifically about the foods you should be eating.

We keep this simple. Don't worry about counting calories or measuring your serving sizes; eat until full. Yes—really! The human body doesn't have any mechanisms for counting calories, so why are so many people meticulously tracking every calorie they consume? You are not a calculator. You are not a math equation. You are a complex chemistry lab, with sophisticated internal "checks and balances."

---

[22] NBC News. https://www.today.com/health/why-fat-your-diet-good-weight-loss-glowing-skin-t102800

There is one caveat that needs mention. This book and the Keto Flex lifestyle are based on the assumption that you eat to provide nourishment for yourself, and not to satisfy a deep emotional need. Personal relationships to food can be very complex, and psychological eating disorders—of all types—are common. These include anorexia nervosa, bulimia, bingeing and/or purging, and simply feeling compelled to eat to alleviate depression or anxiety. If you eat to satisfy a deep-seated emotional compulsion, then no diet or eating plan will change your behavior until you first seek mental health counseling or therapy.

Having said that, let's look at a typical keto meal plan. It's just a suggestion; there are many possibilities! The overall goal is to eat *three meals* that are low in carbohydrates, moderate in protein, and high in wholesome natural fats. If you're the average diurnal (daylight) person, three meals a day is probably going to follow a schedule like this: breakfast at 7:00 AM, lunch at 1:00 PM (six hours later), and dinner at 7:00 PM (six hours later). Then you've got 12 hours until breakfast the next day. Many people get nervous when they think about going 12 hours with no food, but trust me, that's the way your digestive system was designed many thousands of years ago. Those 12 hours are important to clear out your stomach and stabilize your blood sugar. You are giving your body a break from producing insulin every time you eat, which can eventually lead to insulin resistance.

And I'll bet that when you wake up in the morning, you will not feel ravenous; you'll feel normal and clear-headed, ready to enjoy the day.

Clean Keto Vs Dirty Keto

When you conduct a quick search on "Dr. Google" for the keto diet, it will provide you with over 200 million results. It's enough information to confuse the heck out of you. One thing is for sure, there is not one way to do it. Many people who teach keto do not teach it with respect to the body at the cellular level. Yes, there's certain foods that will get you into ketosis, but will they actually help you achieve perfect health?

One of the biggest nuggets of keto research I've come across over the years has been about bad fats. They are bad because they are unstable, rancid fats that cause cellular havoc inside of the body. I remember sitting down for a Keto Kamp Podcast interview, where I currently live in Miami, with MIT research professor Brian Peskin. I asked Brian about these bastardized fats.

I asked him which he believed was worse for our health, these unstable fats or smoking cigarettes?

Being the analytical mind that he has, he said, "Let's look at the research."

If someone smoked two packs of cigarettes every day for 28 years, their chance of developing lung cancer within those 28 years is 16 percent.

Compare that to someone consuming these cooked vegetable oils, every day for 28 years. Their chance of developing cancer and/or heart disease is 86 percent. Yikes!

When interviewing Dr. Cate Shanahan for The Keto Kamp Podcast, I asked her if her research aligns with Professor Peskin's, and she said when you consume these industrial seed oils it raises your risk of disease closer to 100 percent!

This is because these unstable fats offer no value to the body. When these vegetable oils are consumed, they gunk up out cell membranes and integral membrane proteins (receptor sites), which leads to an increase of inflammation. This blocks the communication from our hormones, nutrients, and oxygen. When you have cellular membrane inflammation, toxins cannot get out of the cell and nutrients and hormones cannot get in. This leads to disease that shows up as a symptom. In their groundbreaking book, *PEO Solution: Conquering Cancer, Diabetes and Heart Disease with Parent Essential Oils,* Professor Brian Peskin and Dr. Robert Rowen showed research that on average it took 18 weeks to reverse the negative effect of the incorporation of these unstable fats to the cell membrane. This means 5 minutes of pleasure equals about 5 months of cell membrane dysfunction!

Here's an excerpt from *PEO Solution*:

PESKIN STUDY: "21st Century Warning: 4½ Months to Rid Patients of the Damaging Fish Oil Excess. It takes 18 weeks to reverse the negative effect of the incorporation of EPA / DHA from fish oil into the cell membrane. This four–month time frame is important to understand, as it coincides precisely with the time frame of significant vascular health improvement, that was accelerated by ceasing fish oil use, as shown in the IOWA screening experiment."

Imagine a childhood friend who shows up to your house uninvited. He enters your house and plops himself on your couch, eats your food, makes a mess in your bathroom; and doesn't like for 132 days! This is what you are doing to your cells each time you eat these unstable fats. Yes, these fats will get you in "ketosis," but they will lead to a destructive path.

Based on a groundbreaking 2018 study by F. De Alzaa, C. Guillaume, and L. Ravetti entitled "Evaluation of Chemical and Physical Changes in Different Commercial Oils during Heating," here's a list of the *truly bad* oils you want to avoid on your Keto Flex lifestyle. Keep in mind they are ubiquitous:

• Canola Oil

- Corn Oil

- Soybean Oil

- Cottonseed Oil

- Rice Bran Oil

- Sunflower Oil

- Peanut Oil

- Fish Oil

- Grapeseed Oil

- Refined Palm

- Hydrogenated Oil

- Safflower Oil

Pro tip: When at restaurants, tell the waiter or waitress you're allergic to the above oils and ask them to use a healthier alternative.

There's a huge misconception that smoke point should be the determining factor to whether or not an oil is healthy to cook with; this has been proven to be false. Researchers also found that contrary to popular belief, an oil's smoke point is a very poor marker of its safety and stability as a cooking oil.[23]

---

[23] De Alazza et al. https://actascientific.com/ASNH/pdf/ASNH-02-0083.pdf

Avoid Dirty Polar Compounds

This is arguably the most important factor.

Polar compounds are the potentially harmful compounds produced when an oil breaks down under heat. Toxic by-products such as lipid peroxides and aldehydes are produced, which are consistently linked to serious diseases.

When it comes to your health, the priority is to choose a cooking oil that produces the lowest amount of harmful polar compounds after heating and oxidation.

Keto Flex-Approved Clean Cooking Oils

The following are Keto Flex approved clean cooking oils:

• Coconut oil

• Grass-fed animal fat

• Avocado oil

• Grass-fed butter

• Grass-fed ghee

• Extra-virgin olive oil

• Pasteurized bacon fat

I highly recommend you listen to my full interview with Professor Brian Peskin on The Keto Kamp podcast, episode 45, and the full interview with Dr. Cate Shanahan, episode 178.

One of the best books on this topic is *Deep Nutrition,* by Dr Cate Shanahan.

Dirty Items to Remove During the First Pillar

To give you a head start into the great land of ketosis, I recommend you *remove* the followings dirty items for the entire first pillar (28 days). I've seen this significantly reduce inflammation inside of the body, which leads to better results:

• Spinach (high in oxalates)

• Almonds (high in oxalates)

• Legumes (including peanuts and chickpeas)

• Corn (typically GMO)

• Soy (Organic fermented soy such as natto and tempeh are fine)

• Cow Dairy (Replace with sheep or goat dairy)

• Nightshades (tomatoes, potatoes, goji berries, peppers, eggplant)

Avoid These Dirty Sweeteners

Do not use the following sweeteners, as I've seen them create dysfunction inside the intestinal tract:

• Xylitol

• Maltitol

• Sorbitol

• Acesulfame Potassium

• Mannitol

• Aspartame

• Sucralose

• Saccharine

Keto Flex-Approved Clean Sweeteners

Try these sweeteners:

• Erythritol

• Pure Stevia

• Monk Fruit

• Allulose

• Non-GMO Dextrose

6 Ways to Beat Sugar Cravings on Keto

1. Cinnamon activates your cell receptor sites and wake up your cells by allowing glucose to get into the cell. Cinnamon has been used for over 4,000 years. It is high in antioxidants. #7 ORAC score, antioxidant score. A cinnamon blood sugar study in type 2 diabetics found that whilst definitive conclusions cannot be drawn regarding the use of cinnamon as an antidiabetic therapy, it does possess antihyperglycaemic properties and potential to reduce postprandial blood glucose levels.[24]

Cinnamon for diabetes can help block the activity of several digestive enzymes to slow the absorption of sugar in the bloodstream after a high-carb meal. Cinnamon bark extracts may be potentially useful for the control of postprandial glucose in diabetic patients through inhibition of intestinal α-glucosidase and pancreatic α-amylase.[25]

Many studies have shown that people with type 2 diabetes can experience significant positive effects on blood sugar markers by supplementing with cinnamon extract.[26]

2. Fenugreek. With trace nutrients (iron, manganese, copper) and a variety of antioxidants, fenugreek is a wonderful keto herb. In a study published in the *Journal of Diabetes and Metabolic Disorders*, it was also observed that the control ground had a "4.2 times higher chance of developing type-2 diabetes compared to subjects in the fenugreek group."[27]

---

[24] https://pubmed.ncbi.nlm.nih.gov/19930003/

[25] https://pubmed.ncbi.nlm.nih.gov/21538147/

[26] https://www.ncbi.nlm.nih.gov/pmc/articles/PMC4003790/

[27] https://www.ncbi.nlm.nih.gov/pmc/articles/PMC4591578/?_ga=2.86043224.1183877052.1564951349-942646101.1564951349

3. Cloves. Consuming cloves can help stop sugar cravings as well. In a study, 30 type-2 diabetics were given capsules containing zero, one, two or three grams of cloves each day for a month to observe their serum glucose levels. Researchers of the study suggested that consuming one to three grams of cloves per day is beneficial for type-2 diabetics to better manage their glucose and total cholesterol levels.[28]

4. Ginseng. In several human studies' American ginseng lowered blood sugar levels in people with type-2 diabetes. The blood sugar lowering effect was seen both on fasting blood sugar and on postprandial (after eating) glucose levels. Drink ginseng tea before or after your keto meals.[29]

5. Glutamine. L-glutamine calms the part of your brain that lights up when you experience a sugar/carb craving. It turns out, sugar is as addicting as cocaine, and some say sugar is 8 times more addicting than cocaine. Wow. Take 500mg of l-glutamine powder, up to 3 times each day. Glutamine will help you ween.

6. Sleep! When your sleep suffers, your blood sugars increase. Sleep deprivation can cause you to have the blood sugars of a type 2 diabetic. Yikes.

---

[28] https://www.organicauthority.com/energetic-health/spices-that-naturally-stop-sugar-cravings

[29] https://www.ncbi.nlm.nih.gov/pmc/articles/PMC2781779/

Studies show that even one night of sleep deprivation changes the levels of our hunger and appetite hormones, leading to increased hunger. It also affects the way your brain's motivation centers respond to the sight or thought of food.[30]

I put together my favorite keto and fasting supplements for you at www.ketokampkit.com

For the first 14 days, I recommend you consume 3 meals per day with no snacking in between. Here are some meal examples for you.

Suggested Daily Keto Meal Plan

Breakfast

Choose one:

• 5 Runny, sunny-side-up eggs with half an avocado and arugula, cooked in avocado oil. Sprinkle 2 tablespoons of nutritional yeast.

• Fatty (keto) smoothie consisting of ¾ cup of full-fat coconut milk, ¼ cups of water, half an avocado, 2 full scoops of grass-fed

---

[30] Scientific American. https://www.scientificamerican.com/article/getting-more-sleep-can-reduce-food-cravings/

collagen protein powder, 2 tablespoons of organic raw walnut butter and ice.

(Skip the toast or muffin!)

Lunch

Choose one:

• Fatty salad, with 5-7 cups of green leafy vegetables, 2 tablespoons of extra virgin olive oil, handful of raw macadamia nuts, sea salt, and black pepper. For protein, add a piece of 8 ounces of wild salmon or grass-fed beef.

• Spaghetti squash noodles with sliced free-range chicken (8 ounces), handful of macadamia nuts, and drizzled with extra virgin olive oil.

Dinner

Choose one:

• Half a sweet potato, steamed Brussels sprouts, and two servings of ¼ organic chicken (leg/thigh) with the skin on.

• 8-ounce grass-fed steak, sautéed arugula, and 1 cup steamed Brussels sprouts with 1 tablespoon grass-fed butter on top.

Love Those Bitter Foods

Since we're talking about specific foods, let's take a moment to discuss bitter foods.

It may seem like an esoteric topic, but it's highly relevant to the evolution of the typical diet of people in industrialized nations.

You probably know that over the centuries, we humans have hybridized many foods to make them more palatable, cheaper, or last longer on the shelf. Corn is a good example—the plump, sweet variety you find at the grocery store bears little resemblance to the rugged maize that was first domesticated by native peoples in Mexico about 10,000 years ago. The ancient cob was less than a tenth of the size of modern corn cobs, at about 2 cm (0.8inch) long. It produced only eight rows of tough, colorful kernels, about half that of modern maize.

And squash, which is one of the sweetest vegetables on the menu today, used to be intensely bitter. Back in the Paleo days, wild vegetables were small, stringy, and bitter. But as soon as we humans settled down on farms and turned our attention to agricultural productivity, we started breeding our food to taste better: less bitter, less fibrous, and more carbohydrate-dense. The process of sweetening and de-fibering of our food accelerated as we got better and better at hybridizing, until most people today don't eat anything like the wild vegetables that our ancestors spent so long breeding.

The problem is that the compounds that gave ancient vegetables their bitter taste were also powerful antioxidants that helped protect us against inflammation and chronic disease. By processing bitterness out of our food, we've lost many essential health benefits.

Ever wonder why coffee is so popular? Here's one reason: Coffee is one of the few truly bitter foods remaining in the typical American diet, and it's also one of the few remaining foods rich in antioxidants. In fact, research has revealed that coffee provides up to 45 percent of the antioxidants in typical Western diets. Even though coffee is a small percentage of our total food and beverage consumption, because it's so rich in antioxidants, which is also what make it bitter, that it can account for a large percentage of our antioxidant intake.

These bitter antioxidants provide a wealth of health benefits, especially when they're eaten in keto-friendly foods as part of your regular diet. Research has shown reduced inflammation, improved blood sugar control and insulin sensitivity, better metabolism in fat cells, and reductions in blood pressure. They also support your gut microbiome and may even help protect against cancer.[31]

---

[31] PaleoLeap.com. https://paleoleap.com/bitterness-modern-food/

What to do? The answer is that you can dampen the bitter flavor of many vegetables while keeping the health benefits. You do this by leveraging fat to make delicious recipes full of antioxidant-rich vegetables.

Traditional indigenous diets that cook with vegetables rely upon fat as an essential part of the food preparation process. Studies have shown that the inclusion of fat in the mouth dulls its receptivity to bitter taste. If you eat a kale salad with olive oil or a dish of baked cabbage with bacon fat, you'll register the vegetables as tasting less bitter, but it won't bother you because the bitterness will be moderated by the fat. You'll still get all the benefits of eating the bitter compounds.

The great chef Julia Child, who had no tolerance for fake foods, said, "With enough butter, anything is good." Her love of butter went against the mainstream attitude. Many "experts" preached that that butter led to heart attacks. As usual, Julia Child was ahead of her time. She also reportedly said, "If you don't like broccoli, put more butter on it."

Oh, and if you don't like butter? She had an answer for that: "If you're afraid of butter, use cream."

Bitter foods, including many herbs, leafy greens, ginger, lemons, limes, apple cider vinegar, cacao, and bitter melon, all contain fat-soluble vitamins (A, D, E, and K) as well as liver-boosting nutrients such as sulfur. These are necessary for the body to be able to produce bile, a fluid that is made and released by the liver and stored in the gallbladder. Bile contains water, cholesterol, bile acids (also called bile salts), bilirubin (a breakdown product of old, recycled red blood cells), and other trace elements. It's needed for optimal digestion and to help the liver work at prime level. It breaks down fats into fatty acids, which can be taken into the body by the digestive tract.

For thousands of years, people have used "bitters" as digestive tonics. These have typically included alcohol-based leaves, roots or flowers, and improve digestion after a large meal. There may be solid science to support these beliefs. That's largely because bitters may trigger the production of stomach acid, which facilitates a variety of digestive processes when the food you've eaten makes its way to the intestinal region. Additionally, bitters may increase the production of digestive enzymes, which further aids food absorption.

Five Reasons Why You Can't Get into Ketosis—and the Solutions!

1. Too Many Carbohydrates

In general, most people can achieve ketosis by dropping their total carbohydrates to 50 grams per day.

Keep an eye out for "carbohydrate creep"! With processed foods, it's important to read the ingredients list.

The solution is to drop your carbohydrates to below 20 grams per day. You can use an app like Cronometer to keep track of your carbohydrates. You can find it at www.cronometer.com/ketokamp.

2. Electrolyte Dumping

As you learned earlier when we spoke about the keto flu, electrolytes are key on keto. There's a process called "electrolyte dumping." Carbohydrates are stored in the body with water. Lowering carbohydrate intake leads to increased water excretion and decreased water retention. Less carbs means less insulin release, causing the kidneys to excrete more sodium. Loss of sodium impacts the balance of other key electrolytes.

When you don't replenish electrolytes on keto, this can result in common symptoms when doing keto such as brain fog, the keto flu, and not feeling good on the keto diet.

The solution is for the first 14 days, consume the Keto Kamp Cocktail:

12-16 ounces of water

1-2 tablespoons of apple cider vinegar

1-2 teaspoons of cream of tartar

A pinch or two of sea salt

3. Too Much Fasting, Too Soon

You might be fasting too much, too soon. Fasting is a muscle you want to develop over time. When your body is metabolically inflexible, your brain is dependent on glucose in the form of carbohydrate calories. When you practice fasting before developing metabolic flexibility, it can be a struggle. When glucose gets low in the brain, the brain will send the body intense cravings for carbohydrates in order to fulfill its desire for glucose. You might have a strong willpower to persevere, but your innate intelligence will win this battle because it will start to raise cortisol and glucose, and even break down healthy protein to convert into sugar via gluconeogenesis in order to meet the brain's demand.

The solution is to shorten your fasting window as you build up your metabolic machinery.

4. Poor Sleep and/or Too Much Stress

Yes, too much stress will kick you out of ketosis. When cortisol is high, glucose follows, and ketones drop. There was a recent study in *Scientific American* that showed poor sleep produces higher levels of the stress hormone cortisol, higher levels of glucose, and higher levels of the hunger hormone ghrelin.

The solution is practice one or more of these simple ways to reduce stress:

- Gratitude journaling

- Practice self-love

- Practice loving others

- Get rid of toxic relationships

- Turn off the news!

Don't neglect your sleep. Sleep is the Swiss Army knife of health, and is foundational for achieving perfect health. The topic of sleep is outside the scope of this book, but I recommend you read my book *The Power of Sleep*, and Devin Burke's *The Sleep Advantage* to learn more. I also discuss it more in depth in chapter 11.

5. Toxins

This is the most common reason why people struggle to get into ketosis, or why you keep getting kicked out of ketosis. We live in the most toxic world in the history of humanity. The number one priority for the body is survival. When toxins enter the body via breathing, skin absorption, and eating, the body does not want these toxins to enter vital organs which can potentially kill you. This is why peroxisome proliferator-activated receptor gamma (PPARy) gets activated in the body as a survival mechanism. PPARy takes those toxins and shuttles them into fat cells, and can even create new fat cells for these toxins to live in. This is how toxins make you fat. Why is the body so cruel? It's trying to save your life! When you start your Keto Flex lifestyle, you will be shrinking and burning fat cells. The body can burn fat cells, but it cannot burn toxins. What ends up happening is these toxins get dumped into the bloodstream and re-absorbed. This can lead to not feeling well, but also cellular membrane inflammation. When the membrane is inflamed, insulin will have a challenge delivering glucose into the cell and keeping glucose levels optimal in the bloodstream. The result could be higher glucose and lowered ketones.

The solution is to be consistent with your bitters, as this does have a detoxification affect. You can also do the following for downstream detox support.

- Weekly massages (deep tissue & lymphatic)

- Weekly chiropractor adjustments

- Movement over exercise

- Foam rolling

- Morning stretching / yoga

If you are curious about your toxic load, take my free toxicity quiz to determine your level of toxicity. Visit www.toxicmiami.com.

The 2/2/2/2 Rule

For the first 14 days on your keto journey, I recommend you follow the 2/2/2/2 rule, which will help your body utilize fatty acids for fuel instead of glucose. This rule makes the transition much smoother. Credit goes to my mentor Dr. Daniel Pompa for this one. Every day, consume the following:

2 tablespoons of grass-fed butter or grass-fed ghee

2 tablespoons of coconut oil or MCT oil

2 tablespoons of avocado oil or olive oil

2 teaspoons of sea salt

The question I receive all the time about this rule is, "How do I get all of these fats in one sitting?" You don't—you spread them out with all of your meals. For example, you would use them for cooking oils, salad dressings, dips, and/or to include with your coffee or tea.

To the Next Pillar

The first Pillar—Adapt—should take two weeks. If you need more time, that's fine! We don't want to arouse the ire of your primal brain watchdog. Just keep at it. You'll find that the less carbs and sugars you eat, the less of them you'll want. Even if you cut your carbs in half, you'll be happier and healthier. If you'd like support from me, and a community of like-minded individuals, I encourage you to become of member of The Keto Kamp Academy. As a member, you'll have access to 200+ videos structured in a step-by-step system to master these four pillars. You'll also receive two monthly health coaching calls with me, and a private online group to interact with other Keto Kamp Academy members. This is a great way to get accountability with your Keto Flex Lifestyle. Visit www.ketokampacademy.com to become a member today.

The next Pillar is to experiment with meal skipping. This is what will get your body started on the process of emptying all those freezers full of free energy that you've got stored up.

Chapter 8: Pillar 2—Fast

If you have been successful eating more healthy fats and fewer carbohydrates for two weeks, then congratulations! Your metabolism is surely thanking you for it. If it took you a little longer to get there, that's okay too. After all, you've probably been eating the same way for years or even decades, and that watchdog in your primal brain is accustomed to thinking about the world as being a non-stop conveyor belt of food. So, keep taking baby steps forward! Eat a little less bread every day. Drive past the sugary coffee shop instead of pulling up to the drive-thru window. At night, even if you feel a little bit hungry, go to bed. You'll be able to sleep just fine.

The next step is to experiment by skipping a meal.

Before you panic, think about this: If you've successfully mastered Pillar I, you've already been fasting for 12 hours a day. I didn't want to call it "fasting," but if you don't eat between dinner at 7:00 PM and breakfast at 7:00 AM, you've been fasting. That's why the first meal of the day is called "breakfast." You are literally breaking from your overnight fast.

By the way, you don't need to "break your fast" in the morning by loading up on food. This is a Western tradition that's actually fairly recent in our history. In the Medieval era and before, the morning meal was minimal, and what we call "lunch" was the first meal of the day. In fact, eating early in the day was thought to be a sin associated with overindulgence and gluttony. In many any other cultures—even today—you'd only have coffee and would not break your fast until noon.

By periodically fasting, you'll be re-aligning your digestive system and metabolism to the way we successfully operated for hundreds of thousands of years during the Paleolithic Era, when the *Homo sapiens* species (that's us) were hunter-gatherers. The idea of deliberately planting and harvesting food—what we call the agrarian era—did not enter our brains until the Neolithic Revolution, which started around 10,000 BCE in the Fertile Crescent, the boomerang-shaped region of the Middle East where people first took up farming. Considering that *Homo sapiens* emerged in Africa about 250,000 years ago, that's very recently!

While on this subject, I'd like to make clear that while the Keto Flex Lifestyle mimics the *way* in which our Paleolithic ancestors consumed food—which was intermittently—it does not advocate actually eating *the exact same foods* as our Paleolithic ancestors. The Keto Flex Lifestyle is not about denying the reality of foods that are available today. It's all about enjoying eating delicious foods like butter, which is decidedly not a Paleo food item! Food should be natural and wholesome; it doesn't matter if it happens to be grown on a farm.

In the Paleolithic Era, our ancestors would wake up in the morning with the sunrise (they followed their natural circadian rhythms—no clocks!). Some went out and hunted for the group's next meal, while others went out and gathered nuts, berries, seeds, fruits, roots, and whatever edible foods they came across. Throughout the day, as the hunters pursued their prey, they might have grazed on nuts and berries they found along the way. Sometimes, they couldn't find food to graze on, and so, by necessity, they fasted. Not eating for a day was no big deal—that's just the way life was.

When the body is in an extended fasting state, your old-school wiring kicks in. The primal brain starts to think, "We're famished! We need to find our next meal. I'm going to do everything possible to keep this body working at maximum efficiency, so we can hunt, kill, and eat our next meal, in order to stay alive."

The power of fasting lies not in the mere reduction of calories, but the beneficial hormonal changes. Your body's pituitary gland naturally produces human growth hormone (HGH), or somatotropin, which is a peptide hormone that stimulates growth, cell reproduction, and cell regeneration in humans and other animals.

One of the main benefits comes from reducing insulin, but there are also increases in nor-adrenalin, cortisol, and growth hormone.

Collectively, these are known as the counter-regulatory hormones, since they all serve to increase blood glucose at a time that the body is not getting glucose from food.

Here we focus on human growth hormone (HGH). It helps to regulate body composition, body fluids, muscle and bone growth, sugar and fat metabolism, and possibly heart function. Beginning in middle age, the pituitary gland slowly reduces the amount of growth hormone it produces.

HGH is said to benefit the quality and appearance of the skin. This hormone can help to speed up healing after an injury and repair muscle tissue after exercise. This helps to build muscle mass, boost metabolism, and burn fat. It's said to slow down the aging process and treat age-related diseases. Research supporting these claims is ongoing.

We do know, however, that fasting is a great stimulus to HGH secretion. During fasting, there is the spike in the early morning, followed by regular secretion throughout the day. Researchers led by M.L. Hartman also showed a five-fold increase in HGH in response to a two-day fast.[32]

---

[32] Hartman, et al. https://pubmed.ncbi.nlm.nih.gov/1548337/

Your Fasting Schedule

Now that you have a brief background on intermittent fasting, I want you to implement it into your schedule.

1. Three days x 12 hours. For 3 days, fast for 12 hours each day. An example of a 12-hour fast is when you eat your last meal at 7:00 PM, and don't eat anything until 7:00 AM the following morning.

Boom! There's your 12-hour fast. If you've graduated from Pillar 1, you're probably already doing this. Easy, isn't it?

You can also look at it from the point of view of when you can eat. Another name for this is time-restricted eating (TRE). It means that you eat only within a "window" of a certain number of hours a day. For example, your "eating window" could be from 7:00 AM until 7:00 PM. You eat during that time, and then after 7:00 PM the kitchen closes and does not reopen until 7:00 AM the next morning.

2. Three days x 14 hours. After 3 days of this, widen the fasting window from 12 hours to 14 hours. For example, make your last meal at 8:00 PM, then make the next meal at 10:00 AM the following morning. Do this for another 3 days.

In this case, your TRE window lasts for 10 hours a day. You can eat within those ten hours, but not outside them.

3. Three days x 16 hours. Next, fast for 16 hours. For example, eat your last meal at 8:00 PM, and your first meal at 12:00 noon the next day. When you are able to complete a 16-20 hour fast, three days in a row, you have now unlocked the next step in your journey.

Here, your TRE window is 8 hours.

Three Helpful Hints for Fasting

Unfortunately, many people who practice fasting do not experience the wonderful benefits it has to offer because they give up. Why do they give up? They simply don't know the rules.

There are three things you can do to make intermittent fasting easier so you can accelerate fat loss and increase mental clarity.

1. Get keto adapted. The first way to make intermittent fasting easier for you is to build up your "fasting muscle" by getting keto adapted.

Before we get into that, let's clear up a common point of confusion between the terms "fat adapted" and "keto adapted."

Fat-adapted means your body can convert fat to energy. When you're fat-adapted, you don't need a steady stream of glucose to stay active. Instead, during food deprivation your body can access a ready supply of energy in the form of body fat. Then, after the crisis, you can quickly go back to burning carbs.

Back in Paleolithic times, this adaptation was a necessity. Our distant ancestors didn't have 24/7 food access. When calories became scarce, their fat mass kept them alive, often for extended periods. For example, imagine a Paleolithic hunter-gatherer who weighs 150 pounds with just 10 percent body fat. Do the math. That's 15 pounds of fat, or roughly 60,000 calories he's carrying around—enough to keep him going for more than two weeks. Of course, after periods of deprivation, he's got to eat more to replace the "fat bank" he had accessed. When you're fat-adapted, you can process a load of carbs and then return to burning fat once blood sugar and insulin levels subside.

When the metabolism has the flexibility to shift from burning through its sugar reserves to tapping into fat stores, this accelerates fat loss and the benefits of fasting.
Keto-adapted is slightly different. It means that being in ketosis— burning fat instead of carbs—is the rule rather than the exception. Think of fat-adapted as being the first (and very positive) step toward better health and loss of excess weight, and keto-adapted as the next step.

2. Use crutches! The second way to get better results with fasting is for you to use fasting crutches if you need to. There are certain beverages and food items you can have during a fast and still maximize its benefits. My favorite fasting crutches are tea, coffee, bone broth, and fats.

3. Rethink your "break fast." The third way to make fasting easier is to break the fast with mostly protein and fat; not carbohydrates. As you're exiting a fast, be mindful of your blood sugar, and avoid sharp blood sugar spikes. Immediately following a fast, your body can be very sensitive to carbohydrates, and added sugars or processed carbohydrates could send your insulin spiking through the roof.

Immediately following a fast, you'll probably want to avoid high-lactose dairy. Start with low-lactose dairy products such as butter, hard cheeses, and lactose-free milk.

Healthy staples like broccoli, cauliflower, and Brussels sprouts may make you uncomfortable. These veggies contain plenty of fiber, plus a trisaccharide called raffinose that humans have difficulty digesting. When you're eating normally they're very appropriate, but after fasting they may cause gas and bloating.

When breaking a fast, eat less-starchy, non-cruciferous vegetables cooked in healthy fats (such as avocado oil, grass-fed butter); and protein, avocado, and bone broth.

Science Backs It Up

There is research study evidence showing its many health benefits.

In their 2019 study entitled, "Ten-Hour Time-Restricted Eating Reduces Weight, Blood Pressure, and Atherogenic Lipids in Patients with Metabolic Syndrome," Dr. Pam Taub and others tested a group of subjects who had metabolic syndrome. This means they all showed a cluster of conditions that occur together, including increased blood pressure, high blood sugar, excess body fat around the waist, and abnormal cholesterol or triglyceride levels. Metabolic disorder increases the risk of heart disease, stroke, and type 2 diabetes.

The 19 participants underwent 10 hours of TRE (all dietary intake within a consistent self-selected 10-hour window) for 12 weeks. The researchers found this TRE intervention improved their cardiometabolic health, and concluded, "TRE is a potentially powerful lifestyle intervention that can be added to standard medical practice to treat metabolic syndrome."

Dr. Pam Taub, a cardiologist at the University of California, San Diego's School of Medicine, and an author of the study, said, "We saw a 3 percent reduction in their weight and a 4 percent reduction in abdominal visceral fat." (This was a period of only 12 weeks.) The researchers also found that cholesterol and blood pressure levels improved, sleep quality improved, and many of the participants reported having more energy.

"When you go into a fasting state," Taub explained, "you start to deplete the glucose stores in your body, and you start to use fat as your energy source. You can enter a low-grade state of ketosis."[33]

Remember, these participants did a TRE of 10 hours, with 14 hours of fasting, and they didn't eat a special diet. Imagine the results they—and you—could get with the Keto Flex Lifestyle over a longer period of time!

Even if you don't need to lose weight, intermittent fasting is a health booster! In a 2018 study entitled, "Early Time-Restricted Feeding Improves Insulin Sensitivity, Blood Pressure, and Oxidative Stress Even without Weight Loss in Men with Prediabetes," researchers conducted a supervised controlled feeding trial to determine whether intermittent fasting (IF) had benefits independent of weight loss by feeding participants enough food to maintain their weight. They used early time-restricted feeding (eTRF), a form of IF that involves eating early in the day to be in alignment with circadian rhythms in metabolism. They found that male subjects with prediabetes showed improvements in insulin sensitivity, β cell responsiveness, blood pressure, oxidative stress, and appetite. They demonstrated that

---

[33] Taub, Panda, et al. https://www.cell.com/cell-metabolism/pdfExtended/ S1550-4131(19)30611-4

eTRF improved cardiometabolic health and that IF's effects were not solely due to weight loss.[34]

Lisa's Story

Lisa, age 57, suffered with inflammation and plantar fasciitis. Her podiatrist had given her cortisone shots in both of her feet. This did not help. She told me, "I gained a lot of weight and ended up in a wheelchair. Because of the inflammation, I couldn't move, much less lose weight." She was scared, because both her parents had died of autoimmune disorders, and she thought she was destined for the same fate.

Then one day she was at the gym, taking a water class, when she saw a woman in her early 20s who, despite being large in size, had a tremendous amount of energy. Lisa asked her how she did it, and she replied it was her ketogenic diet. So, Lisa went home and began her research. She found the Keto Kamp Academy, and it clicked with her. "It's been two years," she said, "And wow! What a journey! And it's not just following one plan, it's the flexing." In a matter of months, Lisa went from not even being able to stand up —just lying on her couch—to attending a fundraising event (this was just before the pandemic struck) and dancing the night away to

---

[34] Sutton et el. https://www.sciencedirect.com/science/article/pii/S1550413118302535

an 80s band. For her, it's all about focusing on health from the inside out, because if you take care of your inside, your outside will follow along. The key expression is "upstream cellular heath." If you keep your cells healthy, they will keep you healthy. Today, Lisa is vibrant and full of life—and light on her feet! She told me that she was pleasantly surprised at how young she feels, as if the clock had been turned back.

In some families, the keto diet, or the example of good health that it sets, can be contagious. Lisa's husband Michael did keto with her and loved it. Her children saw the difference it made, and they now eat heathy, low-carb diets and avoid processed foods.

Chapter 9: Pillar 3—Phasing

In the Keto Flex Lifestyle, Pillar 1 called for you to adjust your food choices. Depending on the type of keto diet you've chosen—classic or one of many modified diets—you've cut down on your carbs, modified protein, and increased the amount of healthy fats. This puts less sugar into your system, which causes your body to switch more readily to burning fat for fuel. This process produces ketones, which your cells are happy to use for energy.

To amplify the positive effects of the keto diet, Pillar 2 showed you how to intermittently fast. By ensuring that no food energy is being introduced for at least 12 hours every day—or even up to 16 hours—you're giving your digestive system time to reset, your insulin levels to subside, and for more ketosis to occur. And remember, all of this is without calorie counting or weighing. You just eat normal keto-friendly meals within your time-restricted window of eating.

Now you're ready to enter Pillar 3 and unleash the full power of the Keto Flex Lifestyle.

Let's move up to the carnivore diet.

"The what?" you say. "Carnivore?"

Yes! As you know, the word "carnivore" comes from the Latin "*carn,*" for "flesh." We're talking about meat. Actually, any product that comes directly from a creature that walks, swims, or flies.

For some people, the idea of eating nothing but animal products would be like a dream come true. For others, it might seem gross. Either way, there's a good reason for it.

Now that your body has been introduced to the idea of the keto diet in which you restrict carbohydrates in order to encourage your body to use fat as fuel, and you are comfortable with that, the next step is to *force* your body to rely upon ketones for fuel. This will take your fat-burning power to the next level!

The concept is simple. You cannot starve yourself in order to enter sustained ketosis. It's just not safe—your body needs nutrients. But you can shut off the spigot of carbs, and by consuming only protein and fat, compel your body to live off its ample reserves of stored fat. In the Classic Keto diet, carbs are greatly reduced from the standard diet—you should be eating four units (by weight) of fats, and just one unit each of protein and carbs. So with the Classic Keto diet, you're still getting some carbs, which can be converted by your body into glucose to feed your cells.

The carnivore phase cuts those carbs to *zero*.

Fruits and vegetables have some carbs, so they are out.

Animal products, ranging from fish to steak to eggs, have no carbs, so they are in.

When you think about it, it's pretty logical. And if you take a multivitamin/mineral supplement every day, you're going to get the nutrients you need. By providing your body with zero carbs, and hence zero glucose, while still providing more than enough nutrition to keep you mentally and physically active, your liver will have no choice but to crank out the ketones to keep your cells happy.

If you eliminate carbs, what are you left with? Fat and protein.

That describes a nice juicy ribeye steak!

There are other reasons why you want to periodically cut all carbs from your diet. One of those reasons is "antinutrients."

Antinutrients

Antinutrients are chemicals found in plants that keep your body from absorbing essential nutrients from food. They prevent the body from being the efficient micronutrient sponge that it was meant to be. People and animals pull the nourishment we need from our surroundings, but as evolution would have it, many plants developed the capacity to fight back. Nutrient-sapping phytochemicals protect tasty edibles from being devoured to the point of extinction.

This state-of-the-art defense system taught animals that overconsumption resulted in sickness and sometimes death. Animals either evolved to digest the antinutrient-rich plants, or they stopped eating them.

There are several compounds in the foods we eat classified as anti-nutrients. Antinutrients are found in their highest concentrations in grains, beans, legumes and nuts, but can also be found in leaves, roots and fruits of certain varieties of plants. Examples include:

Glucosinolates in cruciferous vegetables (broccoli, Brussels sprouts, cabbage). These can prevent the absorption of iodine, which may then interfere with thyroid function and cause goiter. Those already with an iodine deficiency or a condition called hypothyroidism are most susceptible.

Lectins are proteins in legumes (beans, peanuts, soybeans), grains, and nightshades that can block the absorption of calcium, iron, phosphorus, and zinc. They stick to your intestinal wall and creating intestinal permeability.

When food moves through your gastro-intestinal tract, it rubs against into your gut's lining, causing microtrauma. Usually, your cells repair those bumps and bruises before they become a problem. Lectins interfere with that process. They adhere to the walls of your gut, preventing repair. The ensuing damage causes low-level inflammation in your GI tract.

When you eat a lot of lectins, your gut wall can develop holes, and its contents can then seep into your bloodstream, causing leaky gut syndrome.

Thousands of varieties of lectins exist in most plant species. Not all of them are toxic or cause intestinal damage. Some plants contain drastically more lectins than other food sources do, which is why wheat, beans, quinoa, peas, peanuts, white potatoes, tomatoes, and eggplants are suspect. The more you eat, the more damage you might be causing to your body. Instead, concentrate on getting most of your nutrients from foods that come with low risk.

Lectin sensitivity varies widely person to person. You might be able to eat lectins morning, noon, and night, and never have a problem, while your friend can't touch the stuff. You'll know you have a problem with lectins if you experience inflammation, brain fog, migraines, stomach issues, acne, or joint pain after eating a lectin-rich meal. The lectins in nightshades, in particular, are a common autoimmune trigger and can cause sensitivities in a lot of people. To test yourself, fill up on a nightshade-heavy lunch—we're talking about tomatoes, peppers, and potatoes—and see how you feel afterward.

Oxalates in green leafy vegetables and tea can bind to calcium and prevent it from being absorbed. Also referred to as oxalic acid, they can be found in plant sources such as fruits, vegetables, nuts and seeds. Oxalate can also be produced naturally by your own body.

Oxalates often bind to minerals such as calcium and are excreted out of the body through the stool. However, high amounts of oxalate can build up in the kidneys, leading to the formation of kidney stones, which occur when hard mineral deposits form within the inner lining of the kidneys, causing symptoms like stomach pain, nausea, and vomiting.

Phytates (phytic acid) in whole grains, seeds, legumes, and some nuts, can decrease the absorption of iron, zinc, magnesium, and calcium. Phytic acid binds to these minerals, preventing their absorption, so you get little nutrition from the food.

Phytate also inhibits the digestive enzymes pepsin, trypsin, and amylase. Trypsin and pepsin are involved in the breakdown of protein, while amylase is required for the breakdown of starch. When those enzymes aren't present in the right amounts, food doesn't get processed properly, and your body misses out on key nutrients.

Think about it like this: If your body has an overload of phytate, while there are fewer nutrients to go around, the body is also substantially less efficient at breaking down macronutrients into their components.

Your body can handle some amount of phytates, but it's a good idea to eliminate the main sources so your minerals will be absorbed. Besides, removing them from your diet completely would be impossible.

To build muscle or burn fat, your body needs a certain amount of protein or carbohydrates. It largely depends on how healthy your gut is. That's because an optimized digestive system requires less food to fuel the body properly.

Gluten is the generic name for proteins found in wheat, rye, barley, and oats. In the digestion of most proteins, the long strands are broken down by digestive enzymes, which cleave or break off groups of amino acids called peptides. The majority of these peptides can be further broken down, absorbed through the intestine, and then transported and used in the body. Gluten is an exception—it cannot be broken down by the digestive enzymes. As a result, it can cause intestinal permeability, or leaky gut.

In terms of how individuals react to the indigestibility of gluten, people fall into two categories: celiac or non-celiac gluten sensitivity. Most of the gluten-sensitive population belong to the latter group, which means they do not test positive for celiac disease, but nonetheless suffer an adverse immune response to gluten, which takes the form of inflammation. Inflammation is generally the culprit behind our gluten-induced brain fog, digestive discomfort, and suboptimal nutrient absorption.

Gluten is hidden in places beyond the obvious sources of bread and pasta. Products like soy sauce, beer, and even processed meats contain gluten that may be downgrading your performance. If you must drink alcohol, then to avoid gluten, skip the beer and reach for potato vodka or gin.

Saponins, also referred to selectively as triterpene glycosides, are bitter-tasting, usually toxic plant-derived organic chemicals that have a foamy quality when agitated in water. In fact, they are produced by plants as a method of natural pest control. Their bitter taste of makes the plant less palatable to birds, insects, and humans.

They are naturally present in quinoa and many other foods, including a wide variety of legumes, vegetables, and herbs. Many people believe saponins irritate the intestinal lining, causing inflammation and all kinds of other trouble.

However, other clinical studies have suggested that saponins can affect the immune system in ways that help to protect the human body against cancers, and also lower cholesterol levels, decrease blood lipids, decrease cancer risks, and lower blood glucose response.

Tannins (or tannoids) are a class of astringent, polyphenolic biomolecules that bind to and precipitate proteins and various other organic compounds including amino acids and alkaloids. Like saponins, plants contain tannins to make themselves unpalatable, and to deter animals from eating a plant's fruit or seeds before they are ripe. Tannins are responsible for that astringent, mouth-coating feeling you get from biting into an unripe pear or plum.

Tannins in tea, coffee, and legumes can decrease iron absorption.

Eating a steady source of antinutrients can lead to gut issues, inflammation, arthritis, and brain fog. Some people are more sensitive to antinutrients than others. You can test your sensitivity with an elimination diet to see if you experience symptoms.

Duration of Pillar 3—Or Any Diet

Readers may wonder, "Why should the Classic Keto Diet advocate for minimal protein, and suddenly in Pillar 3 you're saying we should eat lots of animal protein? Isn't that inconsistent with the first two Pillars?"

The first answer is, "Yes, it's inconsistent."

The second answer is, "No, it's totally consistent."

Confused? No problem! I'll make it clear.

1. It's Inconsistent

Let's discuss the first answer. The inconsistency is deliberate. This is because if you restrict your food choices, it's easy to follow any diet in the short term. But eventually your primal brain will rise up and demand you change. It's incredibly difficult to stick to a diet for months and years. Your brain will scream "No!" and you'll relapse. This is because your primal brain has been hard-wired to expect external conditions to regularly change. Thousands of years ago, variation was the norm. The food supply was inconsistent and varied from season to season. The people who survived under these conditions became the "normal" ones. This relentless adaptation made people stronger, and the primal brain learned that variation was a good thing.

Survival is the #1 priority for the primal brain. It wants to survive, and it will do anything to support that. Major dietary shifts drive survival adaptation mechanisms. To survive changes, the body drives hormonal optimization, making hormones more sensitive and increasing growth hormone. Growth hormone is an anti-aging, healing and fat burning hormone. During this process the body changes its genetic expression and strengthens the microbiome.

Here's the rule: During periods of adaptation, good cells get stronger, while bad cells don't adapt.

We want our cells to get stronger, not sicker.

In our modern industrialized society, where we have all the food we could possibly want, how do make your primal brain happy? *Diet variation* is where the magic happens. I discovered this concept from my health mentor, Dr. Daniel Pompa.

We can mimic the conditions of our ancient existence by forcing changes in our diet. Adapt or die baby! It's a wonderful process. Diet variation is so magical because when you change your diet, your body is forced to adapt. There's not one ancient culture in the history of the world that stuck with one diet their entire life cycle; it just didn't happen.

2. It's Totally Consistent

The reason why Pillar 3 is consistent with the Keto Flex Lifestyle is that it stays absolutely on target to meet the goal of sustained ketosis.

Remember, the foundation of the Keto Flex Lifestyle is to starve your body of carbs that can be turned into glucose. In the absence of glucose, we want the body to activate the ready supply of stored energy in your fat cells. In this way, you'll shed the excess fat and be leaner and healthier. The best way to ease into the Keto Flex Lifestyle is to follow the traditional approach of boosting your fat intake while lowering your consumption of protein and carbs. Once you're accustomed to that approach, to keep your primal brain happy and to take that next step to *zero* carbs, you need to switch it up and shift to a protein-heavy diet. This will keep you feeling full, trick your primal brain into thinking you're adapting to changing conditions, and shut off the supply of carbs, forcing your body to switch to ketones for energy.

Pretty neat, isn't it?

This is why the best timeframe to be following a carnivore diet is 30 to 90 days. You don't do it forever, because the key to success is constant change.

During your 30 days (or more) of carnivore, I recommend you follow a 20/4 intermittent fasting schedule.

20 hours fasting and 4 hours feasting (2 meals)

For example, on your calendar it would look like this:

3:00 PM – 7:00 PM is your eating window. Consume 2 carnivore meals.

7:00 PM – 3:00 PM the next day is your fasted state. Consume only water and sea salt.

Yes, you can change the schedule around based on your lifestyle needs.

One Meal a Day (OMAD)

The more you learn about the keto diet, the more you'll see the acronym OMAD. It stands for "one meal a day."

One of the interesting aspects of the Keto Flex Lifestyle is that instead of feeling like you're starving, which is a feature of most other diets, you're more likely to feel physiologically satiated. When the opportunity to eat presents itself on your schedule, instead of feeling like a happy pig headed for the slop trough to gorge, you're more likely to feel like a finicky housecat who acts like food is a necessary annoyance. (If you've ever owned a cat, you know what I mean!) You won't be going crazy for food.

In my own experience, while on the Keto Flex Lifestyle I generally feel physiologically satisfied, even on one meal a day, but sometimes psychologically unsatisfied. This is simply because eating is a pleasurable experience, and going 23 hours with nothing but water and salt is, well, a little boring at first. But after a while you get used to it, and it seems more like freedom. You don't have to worry about eating or even think about it. You just keep going, like the Energizer Bunny.

The OMAD approach may remind you of the Warrior Diet. Popularized in the book by Ori Hofmekler, the Warrior Diet is based on the idea that ancient warriors had no time to eat because they were too busy rampaging and pillaging, so they ate one big meal before bedtime and then nothing but incidental snacks and water for the following 23 hours. The book shamelessly flatters its readers by proclaiming they can be "predator/victors," and that Hofmekler himself is a magnificent human specimen. I'm sure that's true, but the problem many people have is that the Warrior Diet encourages you to eat during that one meal as much food as you can of any type, and then sleep it off overnight, like a lion sleeps after making a big kill. The challenge is that to get the best results, you need to pay attention to the macronutrient composition of your diet. To improve your body composition and overall health for the better, you need to pay attention to the quality of your diet.

More scientific study is needed on the effects of OMAD. The only research study that I know on OMAD was published in 2007. Entitled "A controlled trial of reduced meal frequency without caloric restriction in healthy, normal-weight, middle-aged adults," for two eight-week periods the researchers allowed the test group to take the Warrior approach and eat the equivalent of three meals in just one meal per day, meaning their total calorie intake over 24 hours was the same as the three-meal-a-day control group. Not unexpectedly, no weight loss was reported.[35]

To verify what I and many other people experience during and after the Keto Flex Lifestyle, we need scientific studies that follow the carefully constructed Keto Flex Diet plan as opposed to the "eat all you can in one sitting" approach.

---

[35] https://pubmed.ncbi.nlm.nih.gov/17413096/

Autoimmune Benefits from the Carnivore Diet

I have Raynaud's autoimmune syndrome. It causes decreased blood flow to the fingers. In some people, it also causes less blood flow to the ears, toes, nipples, knees, or nose. This happens due to spasms of blood vessels in those areas.

The exact cause of Raynaud's is unknown. It is possible that some blood disorders may cause Raynaud's by increasing the blood thickness. This may happen due to excess platelets or red blood cells. Or special receptors in the blood that control the narrowing of the blood vessels may be more sensitive.

If you want to know more about Raynaud's syndrome, just Google it, and look at some of the photos. It can be rather mild or really gross and nasty!

As for me, I would get a flare-up after eating a meal, and my fingers would get swollen, red, and inflamed.

During my 40-day carnivore diet, I only had two small flare-ups. It seemed amazing! As emerging evidence suggests, carnivore has profound benefits on healing the gut.

Raynaud's syndrome is just one of many modern syndromes that seem to plague industrialized nations. From chronic fatigue syndrome to irritable bowel syndrome, we seem to have a global problem with autoimmune disorders. According to the National Institutes of Health, over 23 million people in the United States alone are diagnosed with autoimmune disease, while millions more suffer undiagnosed.

In response, doctors prescribe medicine cabinets full of pharmaceuticals, each one aimed at suppressing a particular group of symptoms. This approach often makes things worse, as a host of side effects mingle with the already debilitating symptoms.

While clinical research on the subject needs to be done, there's growing anecdotal evidence that the carnivore diet has a positive effect on autoimmune diseases including Raynaud's syndrome. In fact, "meat heals" has become a popular tagline within the carnivore diet community. There is a theory that some people— perhaps myself included—have an extreme or allergic reaction to the common plant toxins, including saponins and tannins, which we've discussed in this chapter. So, it's not the fact that animal products have some magical healing property; it's that they *don't* have the toxic compounds that can make some people sick. So if you suffer from a stubborn autoimmune disease that defies a cure, why not follow the carnivore diet for a few weeks? You may get surprising results.

The 4 Keys to Success on Carnivore

Here are the four keys to success when using the Pillar #3 carnivore diet plan.

1. Maintain a 2:1 fat to protein ratio

Instead of the Classic Keto 4:1 ratio of fat to protein, double the amount of protein while keeping the fat. Carbs must be zero.

You can use an app such as Cronometer to track this. Visit www.cronometer.com/ketokamp.

2. Methionine vs glycine ratio

Methionine and glycine are amino acids. Along with 20 other amino acids, they make up the structure of proteins. Methionine is commonly found in muscle meat, while glycine is in animal protein collagen, found in connective tissue, tendons, ligaments, skin, cartilage, and bones.

Methionine is a carrier of methyl groups. When you have too much methionine, it uses up your body's glycine to buffer up the methyl groups. This will mess up your biochemistry.

Glycine balances methionine and helps the amino acid ratio. If you are glycine deficient, it will be difficult to make collagen and glutathione, meaning you may feel sick.

3. Supplements Are Key

Here are three supplements that can make a big difference with your carnivore results.

- Boron (glycinate)

- Bone broth powder

- Organ meat complex

4. If You Are Not Feeling Well on Carnivore:

- You may be eating meat that is very lean. Increase your healthy fats!

- Add raw honey around exercise time and/or before sleep

Tara's Story

Tara started keto one autumn when she was training for a marathon and she hurt her ankle. she was already gluten-free and dairy-free, but a friend suggested she try my keto diet. "At first," she told me, "I wasn't sure I'd like it because I was a runner, but when I tried it, I discovered that it wasn't difficult at all. In fact, I started sharing it with my kids!" For Tara, the water fasting made a big difference. "After the water fast," she said, "I noticed I had much more energy." She did the keto diet, and added fasting on top of it, and saw tremendous results.

Like many people who join the Keto Kamp Academy, Tara initially met with some resistance from her social circle. Her younger sister was a competitive swimmer, and when Tara told her she was going to adopt the keto diet, her sister said, "Are you crazy? You can't run and be athletic on that diet." But Tara was very patient, and as she got results, her sister slowly came around. "If you show the naysayers how much more energy you have," she told me, "and how good you feel, you'll gain their respect. It's all about being focused on good health."

When she began fasting, she was surprised at how easy it was to forgo food. She'd give her kids lunch, and they would say, "Aren't you eating?" and she'd say, "Oh, I'll get something later." Then before she knew it, it would be five o'clock, and she'd have lots of energy and wasn't feeling like she was deprived. To date, the longest water fast she's done was over 61 hours (that's about 2 ½ days), and it was no problem to complete.

Chapter 10: Pillar 4—Flex

Consuming a low amount of carbohydrates over the long term is a good thing. It will cause you to burn excess body fat and improve your overall health.

But there's one important caveat.

A constant, unrelenting state of ketosis—in which your body is burning its own fat for fuel—is obviously unsustainable, because eventually you'd have no more fat. In this chapter, we move into the Flex pillar, which will allow you to maintain your Keto lifestyle month after month, year after year.

Four Reasons Why Prolonged Ketosis Is Counterproductive

My mantra is, "Lose the excess fat; treasure the necessary fat."

Ketosis is a brilliant strategy for accomplishing the first goal.

As for the second goal, prolonged ketosis doesn't have an automatic shut-off valve. If you remain in state of constant ketosis, burning your own fat, then your body will keep doing that as long as it must to stay alive. If necessary to preserve life, once your fat is gone, various bodily functions will be shut off or minimized. This process of shutting down will continue until Mr. Death knocks on your door and says, "Sorry, buddy—time's up."

No one wants that.

To ensure that you're well informed, let's review some of the bad things that can happen if you go too far with ketosis.

1. Fat Burning Slows Down

As levels of body fat drop, your primal brain, whom we thought we had trained to accept a high-fat diet and fasting, will be aroused and will begin to object.

Why and when will this happen?

Your primal brain, that eternal watchdog, will sense that your reserves of fat are becoming depleted. Remembering those long periods of deprivation thousands of years ago, your primal brain will sound the alarm: *The fat supply is running low!*

It will issue the command that your body must preserve its precious fuel. In response, your body will actually slow down fat burning—all for the sake of survival!

When you stay in ketosis too long, the body starts to rebel, and conserve its fuel. A good analogy is if you lived out in the woods and you had stored 500 logs of firewood to heat your cabin for the winter. These were your reserves, because you could still go out and chop more firewood. So if you had to dip into these reserves, you wouldn't be worried.

But now it's early March, and snow still covers the ground. It's been a tough winter and you haven't harvested many trees, and you see that you've got only 50 logs left. That's a very low supply! Suddenly you're reluctant to use them because you don't want to run out. When you had 500 logs, you didn't care about burning them.

The same thing happens with your body fat. This is why when you stay low carbohydrate for too long, your body will *slow down* fat metabolism.

And you know what? This is a good thing. There is a big difference between losing *excess* fat and losing *all* your fat. You want to lose excess fat. But your body needs a small amount of fat, and your primal brain is smart to insist that you meet this minimal requirement.

2. Thyroid Problems

Hormone production is often a function of a "chain of command," as orders are passed from one organ to another, until the desired outcome is achieved. The hypothalamus and the pituitary gland, which are located in the brain, help control the thyroid gland, a butterfly-shaped gland located at the base of your throat, just below the Adam's apple.

To provide their direction to the thyroid, the hypothalamus releases thyrotropin-releasing hormone (TRH), which stimulates the pituitary gland to release thyroid-stimulating hormone (TSH). When the hypothalamus and pituitary are working normally, they respond when:

• Thyroid hormone levels are low, so they secrete more TRH and TSH, which stimulates the thyroid to make more hormones.

• Thyroid hormone levels are too high, so they secrete less TRH and TSH, which reduces hormone production by the thyroid.

The thyroid gland uses iodine from food to make two thyroid hormones: triiodothyronine (T3) and thyroxine (T4). The primary secretory product is inactive thyroxine (T4), which is a prohormone of triiodothyronine (T3). T4 is converted to T3 peripherally by tissues with high blood flow, including the liver and kidneys. In the brain, T4 is converted to active T3 by type 2 deiodinase produced by glial cells.

The thyroid stores T3 and T4, and releases them as they are needed. These two thyroid hormones function in almost every cell in your body, and play a fundamental role in regulating your metabolism and maintaining your resting energy expenditure—that is, the energy you burn just to keep functioning while sitting on the sofa.

Diet can influence thyroid hormone levels, and prolonged ketosis and severe calorie restriction can lead to reduced thyroid function, or hypothyroidism, which is a mechanism to ensure survival in response to perceived famine. The goal is to slow metabolism, preserve energy, and preserve vital organs.

T4 is the inactive form of thyroid, it needs to be converted to T3 which is the active form used by the cells. Do you know which hormone helps with this conversion? Insulin.

Low thyroid hormones cause a drop in levels of insulin, the hormone needed to transport sugar from the blood to different cells throughout the body. Chronic low insulin levels slow down cellular function, including muscle contractions and basic brain function. Over longer periods of time, low insulin levels compromise this T4 to T3 thyroid hormone conversion.

3. Testosterone Deficiency

Sex hormone binding globulin (SHBG) is a protein made by your liver. It binds tightly to three sex hormones found in both men and women—estrogen, dihydrotestosterone (DHT), and testosterone. SHBG carries these three hormones throughout your blood.

SHBG controls the amount of testosterone that your body tissues can use. Too little testosterone in men and too much testosterone in women can cause problems. Factors such as sex, age, obesity, liver disease, and hypothyroidism can change the level of SHBG in your blood. Hypothyroidism is when your thyroid produces an insufficient amount of thyroid hormones, which can happen with prolonged ketosis. What I've seen reviewing lab work over the years is too much SHBG leads to lower testosterone levels, and not enough SHBG leads to an increase in estrogen; both can be problematic for men and women. Long term ketosis can lead to either of these.

4. Leptin Reset

Leptin is your "stop eating!" hormone that plays an instrumental role in your hunger and weight management. It comes from the Greek word *"leptos,"* meaning "thin."

Fat cells produce leptin in proportion to levels of body fat: the more fat cells you have, the more leptin they make. When your body fat increases, your leptin levels go up. Your brain senses the increase in leptin, and thinks, "Okay, we've got enough fat in reserve, so we can stop eating." Thus, you eat less and burn more. Conversely, when you don't eat, your body fat decreases, leading your leptin levels to drop. Your brain, sensing a shortage of leptin, thinks, "Hmm, we're low on fat reserves. Better find some food!" At that point, you eat more and burn less.

This negative feedback loop is similar to the control mechanisms for many physiological functions, such as body temperature, breathing, and blood pressure.

A properly working leptin system tells your brain that you have enough energy stored in your fat cells to engage in normal, everyday metabolic processes. It leads to better brain function, memory, metabolic performance, mental sharpness, and coordination, and it can even affect the regulation of mood and emotion.

This is wonderful—except that many overweight people suffer from *leptin resistance*. They have plenty of blood leptin, but the brain doesn't recognize it. Despite the abundance of leptin, the brain thinks there is too little leptin—and orders the body to *keep eating!*

This is obviously a bad situation. What can cause it?

Several potential mechanisms behind leptin resistance have been identified.

• Free fatty acids. Having elevated free fatty acids in your bloodstream may increase fat metabolites in your brain, and interfere with leptin signaling.

• Inflammation. Inflammatory signaling in your hypothalamus could be a cause of leptin resistance.

• Having consistently high leptin. It may be that your brain gets accustomed to a constant flood of leptin churned out by your fat cells, and becomes "numb" to it.

So, what happens when you follow a low-carb keto diet that puts you in long-term ketosis? Perhaps paradoxically, many people do not suffer from an increase in appetite, as you might expect from falling levels of leptin.

It's complicated, but the short version of the story is that leptin levels will drop, which would normally signal your brain to start eating. But something else happens—your brain becomes more sensitive to the effects of leptin, so a smaller amount of leptin packs more punch.

In addition, the brain's response to leptin is inhibited by inflammation, resulting in increased leptin resistance. Obesity increases inflammation, which increase the brain's "numbness" to high levels of leptin. Inflammation is dramatically reduced by sustained nutritional ketosis. The reduction in leptin resistance due to reduced inflammation adds to the brain's heightened sensitivity to leptin. In other words, on a well-formulated ketogenic diet the brain perceives a *greater* satiety response to *less* leptin. This explains the paradox as to why we see a decrease in appetite with nutritional ketosis.

In order to achieve a sustained state of ketosis, you need to occasionally boost your levels of leptin and send the signal to your brain that higher levels of leptin are normal, and that you need to keep eating. This is another reason why the "flex" part of Keto Flex Lifestyle is so important. We never want your brain to think you're starving—but we also don't want it to forget about eating!

The Value of Protein

Many people who first learn about the Keto Flex Lifestyle assume that because the diet initially calls for a reduction in protein (it's often called a "condiment" rather than an "entrée," that the Keto Flex Lifestyle is anti-protein, or that protein is bad for you. They also cite many other objections to eating protein, all of which are easily dismantled.

Here are some common myths about glucose and protein, which I'm happy to debunk.

Myth #1: The Body and Brain Need Dietary Glucose to Function

This is false. You don't need to consume glucose from carbohydrates in your diet. The fact is your body *makes* glucose. Your own body fat combined with amino acids from the proteins you eat keep blood sugars at homeostasis. The body uses insulin to tightly control blood sugar levels, so that at any given time, less than one little teaspoon of sugar is in your entire bloodstream.

As *Textbook of Medical Physiology* reveals, even after five weeks of complete starvation, and drinking only water, blood glucose levels in the average healthy adult will remain stable. We get all the sugar we require by burning our excess body fat and from the protein we eat. The medical term is *gluconeogenesis*. This is the metabolic process by which organisms produce sugars (glucose) for catabolic reactions from non-carbohydrate precursors.

Substrates (the substances being observed in a chemical reaction) for gluconeogenesis may come from any non-carbohydrate sources that can be converted to pyruvate or intermediates of glycolysis. For the breakdown of proteins, these substrates include glucogenic amino acids (although not ketogenic amino acids). Proteins are a source of gluconeogenic substrates, which under fasting or a low-carbohydrate intake can be used to produce glucose. High-protein (HP) diets are generally low in carbohydrates and assumed to promote postprandial gluconeogenesis.

Excess amino acids from digested protein must be oxidized as fuel or converted into other storage products. The excess ingested protein can, through the process of gluconeogenesis, produce glucose. This would mean that 100 grams of protein could produce about 50 grams of glucose. This should not kick you out of ketosis since the glucose produced will refill your glycogen stores (sugar reserves) found in your liver and skeletal muscle.

Myth #2: Increasing Protein and Fat Will Put You at Risk for Heart Disease

Science is showing us that it's not protein that leads to heart disease, it's the other stuff that we eat that can clog our arteries.

Protein—or more precisely, the amino acids your body needs to make its own protein molecules—come from two sources, animals and plants.

Not all proteins are created equal. Although animal products contain all nine essential amino acids, nuts (including almonds and cashews) and seeds (like sunflower and pumpkin seeds) do not. As a result, they cannot be categorized as complete protein examples.

Your body actually needs essential amino acids in complete protein sources in order to grow and repair tissue.

Here are some good sources of protein from plants:

Nuts and seeds. My favorite keto sources are almonds, cashews, pistachios, walnuts, pili nuts, macadamia nuts and pecans.

Flaxseeds are high in protein, as are chia seeds and pumpkin seeds.

Studies suggest that people who eat nuts regularly are less likely to die of heart disease than those who rarely eat them. This may be because if you fill up on nuts, which are good for you and have no sugar, you're less likely to be eating sugary, carb-laden snacks.

Legumes (beans and peas). If it grows in a pod, it's a legume. These include green beans, black beans, pintos, Lima beans, split peas, garbanzos, and many more. The ubiquitous soybean comes in many forms, including fresh whole green beans (edamame), tofu, and soy milk. Most soy is genetically modified and estrogenic, so I tend to avoid them unless it's organic tempeh and natto. Like nuts, eating beans has been linked to a lower risk of heart disease. You don't have to eat them plain; most people consume legumes in salads, soups, stews, or bean-based dips such as hummus.

Here are your best bets for protein from animals:

Dairy products (milk, yogurt, and cheese). Protein leaders by weight include cheese (real cheese, not that processed crap in a can), cottage cheese, Greek yogurt, cream cheese, and whole milk. Choose full-fat products with no added sugar (be careful with yogurts, which often come loaded with fruity, sugary sweeteners, and are more like liquid candy.) Most studies show no link between heart disease risk and dairy products, regardless of milk fat levels. The worst choices are "low-fat" dairy products that include added sugar. Remember, it's the fat that makes you feel satiated. If you replace the fat with quickly metabolized sugar, in no time you'll be famished again. When choosing dairy, sheep and goat dairy is much better for the body than cow.

Fish and shellfish. Fatty fish such as salmon are a good way to get protein plus heart-healthy omega-3 fatty acids, and studies suggest that people who eat fish have fewer heart attacks than those who avoid it. High-protein fish choices include Alaskan sockeye salmon, wild

Atlantic salmon, sardines, Albacore tuna, tilapia, halibut, and flounder. Most types of shellfish have approximately the same amount of protein as other types of fish and meat. Top choices include clams, shrimp, mussels, and scallops.

Eggs. As one of the most nutritious foods you can find, eggs are a key ingredient in any low-carb diet. They're packed with nutrients that boost health and contain almost zero carbs. For the most benefit, eat the whole egg—both yoke and white. Yolks have nearly as much protein as egg whites, and the yolk is the home of nearly all of an egg's fat content.

Meat and poultry. Meat and poultry are powerful sources of protein. They also provide many other nutrients your body needs, like iodine, iron, zinc, vitamins (especially B12) and essential fatty acids. Protein leaders include bacon, beef, chicken, ham, and pork. Meat contains zero carbs.

Insects. Yep, I'm talking about bugs. In many parts of the world, roasted and toasted insects are part of the everyday diet, and are slowly finding acceptance in industrialized nations.

The average insect—cricket, mealworm, grasshopper—is around half protein by dry weight, with some insects (such as locusts) up to about 75 percent protein. This means that insects are comparable to other animal protein sources, without many of the other nutritional and environmental problems of factory-farmed livestock, including overuse of growth hormones and antibiotics. Insects are incredibly inexpensive to raise, and they don't transmit any viruses to humans. They can be raised in urban environments, on a small footprint.

Currently in America, insect protein is showing up in the form of flours. High-protein insect flour—typically made from crickets —has a nutty flavor that lends itself well to baked goods. Innovative home cooks are using insect flour as a way to fortify the nutritious content of the food without sacrificing flavor, texture or consistency. It can even be used in gluten free and paleo recipes.

Taste's change. It wasn't so long ago that lobster was known as "the cockroach of the sea," a trash food fit to be eaten by only the poorest people. Today it's on the menus of five-star restaurants. Insect products will not be far behind!

The Flex Solution: Feast Days

What can you do to reassure your primal brain that you aren't going to starve to death? You give it a little of what it wants—you give it a *feast day!* Hence the term "Keto Flex." The "flex" part is very important.

I love keto flexing because you teach your body to have hormone flexibility, as well as to be able to switch back and forth between burning fat and glucose. Remember, while in our industrialized culture we have to make a conscious effort to follow such a diet plan, for hundreds of thousands of years our ancestors didn't have to make a conscious effort because this was normal life. Food was available intermittently, and fasting wasn't "fasting," it was just those regular periods during which no food was available, or it had to be rationed. They didn't think about it, they just did it. If you had killed a deer and you knew that deer had to feed your family for a month, would you eat the whole thing in one week? Of course not. You'd smoke the meat, and then dole it out a little bit at a time.

Eating/Fasting Schedules

Here are a few eating/fasting schedules that you can follow. See which one works for you or vary them! All that matters is that you shut off the food spigot on a regular basis for an extended period of time—at least 12 hours, but even for 16 or 24 hours.

Weekly 5-1-1

Credit goes to my health mentor, Dr. Daniel Pompa, for teaching me this method.

This method is a good approach if you've achieved your ideal body weight, or if you want to put on healthy weight.

• 5 days of intermittent fasting for 16 to 20 hours. When you are eating during the 4- to 8-hour window, stick to a ketogenic (high healthy fats) approach. Eat less than 50 grams of carbohydrates and less than half your body weight in protein.

• 1 day, complete a 24-hour water-only fast (dinner to dinner).

• 1 day, complete a feast day. Have three meals of high (healthy) carbohydrates and/or protein. Consume between 100 - 150 grams of healthy carbs and/or protein. Eat less fat on this day.

Weekly 4-2-1

This method is good if you still have 5 to 20 pounds to lose.

• 4 days of intermittent fasting for 16 to 20 hours. When you are eating during the 4- to 8-hour window, stick to a ketogenic (high healthy fats) approach. Eat less than 50 grams of total carbohydrates and less than half your body weight in protein.

• 2 days complete a 48-hour water-only fast.

• 1 day, complete a feast (flex) day. Have three meals of high (healthy) carbohydrates and/or protein. Consume 100 – 150 grams of healthy carbs. Eat less fat on this day.

Weekly 3-3-1

This method is good if you still have 20 or more pounds to lose.

• 3 days of intermittent fasting for 16 to 20 hours. When you are eating during the 4- to 8-hour window, stick to a ketogenic (high healthy fats) approach. Eat less than 50 grams of total carbohydrates and less than half your body weight in protein.

• 3 days complete a 72-hour water-only fast.

• 1 day, complete a feast (flex) day. Have three meals of high (healthy) carbohydrates and/or protein. Consume 100 – 150 grams of healthy carbs. Eat less fat on this day.

16/8 Method

Known as the Leangains protocol and popularized by fitness expert Martin Berkhan, the 16/8 method involves restricting your daily eating window to 8–10 hours and fasting every day for 14 to 16 hours.

Within the daily eating window, you can eat as much as you want, as long as you're eating a ketogenic diet. This method won't work if you eat junk food or an excessive number of calories.

Doing this method of fasting can be as simple as not eating anything after dinner, skipping breakfast, and making lunch your first meal of the day.

The 5:2 Diet

Also called the Fast Diet, and popularized by British journalist Michael Mosley, the 5:2 Diet involves eating normally 5 days of the week. For the other two days of the week—it could be any nonconsecutive two days, like Monday and Wednesday, or Tuesday and Friday—you restrict your food intake to no more than 600 calories per day. On the fasting days, it's recommended that women eat 500 calories and men 600, but it all depends on your level of physical activity.

Alternate-Day Fasting

In alternate-day fasting, you fast every other day. A full fast every other day can seem extreme, so it's not recommended for beginners. You may go to bed very hungry several times per week, which is challenging and probably unsustainable in the long term. Therefore, some of versions allow about 500 calories during the fasting days.

Eat-Fast-Eat

This diet, popularized by fitness expert Brad Pilon, involves a 24-hour fast two or three times per week. Basically, you eat one day, fast the next day, and eat on the third day. Then you repeat the pattern—eat, fast, eat. Water, coffee, and other zero-calorie beverages are allowed during the fast, but no solid foods are permitted.

Because each week has an odd number of days, the eating/fasting days of the week will rotate. If you fast on Tuesday and Friday of the first week, then on the second week you'll fast on Monday, Thursday, and Sunday.

By fasting from dinner one day to dinner the next day, this amounts to a full 24-hour fast. You can also fast from breakfast to breakfast or lunch to lunch—the end result is the same. But you need to be consistent, and fast for a full 24 hours each time.

The Warrior Diet

Mentioned earlier in this book, the Warrior diet advocates eating small amounts of raw fruits and vegetables during the day, followed by one huge meal at night, within a four-hour eating window. This approach is based on the evidence that your body burns fat while you sleep, so if you consume 2,500 calories in a day, you're better off doing it all before bedtime, and then sleeping for at least seven hours.

Random Meal Skipping

This is another approach, and probably the least effective of all of them. Here, you simply skip an occasional meal, such as when you don't feel hungry or are too preoccupied to cook and eat.

If you don't feel hungry one day, skip breakfast and eat a healthy lunch at noon, and then dinner at 7:00PM. That would give you a 16-hour fast from your previous dinner at 7:00 PM.

Skipping one or two meals when you feel inclined to do so is basically a spontaneous intermittent fast. But you must be serious about it, and set goals for yourself. If you assume there are 21 meals per week (7 times 3), then you'd better make sure you skip at least six of them, to equal two fasting days.

Remember, what you eat at meals is extremely important. While you want to consume some carbs to maintain a supply of fat cells and ensure your body can switch back and forth between burning fat and glucose, a diet of crappy, sugary, processed foods will destroy the progress you've made. To stay healthy, eat healthy!

Shannon's Story

Shannon enrolled into my Keto Kamp Academy in October 2019. When she embarked on her journey of healing, she was taking insulin to manage her type 2 diabetes. She completed the first pillar (Adapt), and then decided to make a doctor's appointment. In less than 40 days, Shannon was able to get off her insulin medication. Her doctor also shared that her cholesterol, liver, and kidney function all improved. A side effect of her getting healthy was that she shed 35 pounds of body fat.

Chapter 11: The Healing Power of Sleep

"The best bridge between despair and hope is a good night's sleep." — E. Joseph Cossman

No discussion of the Keto Flex Lifestyle plan would be complete without getting into the critical role of sleep.

Let's dispose of one stupid myth right away: Among certain groups of self-aggrandizing businesspeople, getting by on four hours of sleep a night is taken as a sign of manliness or high achievement. The naïve logic goes like this: Because you're not being *visibly productive* while you sleep, it therefore must be *wasted time*. Sleep is nothing, and if you sleep more than a few hours a night, you are lazy.

Anyone who knows anything about the human brain knows this is dangerous nonsense. Sleep is vital to brain health, and sleep deprivation is a significant health risk.

Keep Your Brain Healthy

In our industrialized, hypercompetitive culture, sleep deprivation is such a chronic condition these days that you might not even realize you suffer from it. Science has revealed that short, interrupted, or impaired sleep can:

• Dramatically weaken your immune system.

• Accelerate tumor growth—tumors grow two to three times faster in laboratory animals with severe sleep dysfunctions.

• Cause a pre-diabetic state, making you feel hungry even if you've already eaten, which can wreak havoc on your weight.

• Seriously impair your memory. Even a single night of poor sleep—meaning sleeping only 4 to 6 hours—can impact your ability to think clearly the next day.

• Impair your performance on physical or mental tasks, and decrease your problem-solving ability.

Let's take a closer look at the brain.

Sleep is when your brain does its housekeeping. While you sleep, your brain is literally doing millions of processes every microsecond. New brain cells are getting produced. New connections are being made.

While you sleep, your brain processes information it received while it was awake. As the author John Steinbeck wrote, "It is a common experience that a problem difficult at night is resolved in the morning after the committee of sleep has worked on it."

Here are two more pithy observations about the beauty of sleep:

"Each night, when I go to sleep, I die. And the next morning, when I wake up, I am reborn." — Mahatma Gandhi.

"Sleep is the best meditation."— Dalai Lama.

While awake and asleep, your brain consumes huge amounts of glucose and oxygen. As a result of all of these processes, waste products are created. For these it requires its own detoxification system, which is run by the glial cells. This system has been called the glymphatic system. Glymphatic transport results in the collection of waste products, such as metabolites and proteins, and their transfer to the cerebrospinal fluid, which carries them out of the brain to sites where the cerebrospinal fluid drains.

Because it goes to work "after hours," this system is ten times more active when you are asleep than when you are awake.

Our brain cells actually shrink up to 60 percent to make more room for cleaning itself. This is huge. It's not just about getting more sleep to have more energy. Your brain is breaking down rapidly if you are not getting high-quality sleep.

Look at the devastation of Alzheimer's disease. This is the inability of the brain to clean itself. It's the buildup of waste products, and the brain's inability to "clean house" that leads to problems. When brain waste and toxins build up due to lack of sleep, we think less clearly. Memory is disrupted, stress hormones aren't cleared, immunity is lowered, anxiety and depression increase, and neurogenesis is slowed.

Only now are we beginning to understand just how important sleep is to health and rejuvenation. The brain literally renews itself during sleep via neurogenesis and deep cleansing. Making a good night's sleep a priority can change your life in more ways than you realize.

Burn Fat While You Sleep

There's more. *Good sleep also helps you lose excess fat.* I love it when I'm asked to give one simple and effective tip that can transform someone's health and break through any fat loss plateau. What I'm about to talk about is so simple, it's amazing and genius once you understand it.

If your goal is to lose fat, but nothing seems to work, your first step is to start with your sleep. I believe fixing your sleep should come before changing your diet or working out at the gym.

You burn most of your fat during the night, not during the day. In fact, 98 percent of fat burning takes place during sleep.

How the heck is this possible?

It's all about your hormones.

When it comes to fat loss, it is all about the hormones, baby.

Hormones are the language of the human body. They are chemical messengers within the cells of our body; we have over 600 of them! Hormones are the reason why your arms are the same length, why you can turn food into fuel, and why you changed from head to toe at puberty.

Your body and your hormones are designed to communicate with each other efficiently to achieve a common goal: to function normally. When you are functioning normally, you are thriving. Food is used for fuel, energy levels are superb, and you feel like you are firing on all cylinders. When our hormones are not able to effectively communicate, symptoms (weight gain) and disease states occur.

Let's say you have a group of hormones. We'll call them testosterone. Your testosterone hormones are located in Florida; they are attempting to communicate with your thyroid hormone, which is located in California. Testosterone is sending the message, "Yo, thyroid. We are going to meet in New York at 9:00 PM with the rest of the hormones to process a meal and turn it into fuel." If our cell membranes have a dysfunction, and our hormones are not balanced, these hormones are unable to effectively communicate with each other. Therefore, thyroid never gets the message. Thyroid ends up in Canada a day late, freezing its ass off. Poor thyroid. The meal is then not used as fuel and is instead stored as fat.

The bottom line is this: if your hormones aren't able to communicate effectively, you will have problems with energy, fat gain, and much more.

Okay, so what has the biggest influence on your hormones? Sleep!

You go through four cycles of sleep. For most people—depending on your own circadian rhythm—growth hormone spikes between midnight and 2:00 AM. Growth hormone is a fat burning and anti-aging hormone. If you are going to bed past midnight, you may be missing this hormonal wave. You can catch the next one, but you are already a step behind.

Here are the six most fat-burning hormones:

1. Triiodothyronine (T3). Made by the thyroid gland, T3 and T4 work together to regulate how your body uses energy. These hormones also play an important role in controlling your weight, body temperature, muscle strength, and nervous system.

2. Growth hormone, or somatotropin, also known as human growth hormones in its human form, is a peptide hormone that stimulates growth, cell reproduction, and cell regeneration.

3. Insulin-like growth factor 1 (IGF-1), also called somatomedin C, is a hormone similar in molecular structure to insulin, which plays an important role in childhood growth and has anabolic effects in adults.

4. Glucagon is a peptide hormone, produced by alpha cells of the pancreas. It works to raise the concentration of glucose and fatty acids in the bloodstream, and is considered to be the main catabolic hormone of the body.

5. Testosterone is most often associated with the male sex drive, and plays a vital role in sperm production. It also affects the way men store fat in the body, red blood cell production, and bone and muscle mass.

6. Adrenaline, also called epinephrine, is a hormone released by your adrenal glands and some neurons. Also known as the "fight-or-flight hormone," it's released in response to a dangerous, stressful, exciting, or threatening situation. Adrenaline helps your body react more quickly by making the heartbeat faster, increasing blood flow to the brain and muscles, and stimulating the body to make sugar to use for fuel.

Sleep deprivation is also linked to insulin resistance, a slowed down metabolism and an increase in appetite.

Two hormones in particular have a big effect on weight: leptin and ghrelin. When you're sleep-deprived, there's a 20 percent increase in the hunger hormone, ghrelin. To compound the problem, levels of leptin, the hormone that tells you that you are full, drop when you are sleep deprived. This increases your appetite and hunger.

Wait, there's more. *Cravings*. When you're sleep deprived, your cortisol level increases. Your brain doesn't like it when your cortisol is high for extended periods of time. So, the front part of the brain communicates to the back part of the brain, and says, "We need to do something to lower this cortisol." How does the body do this? By eating high carbohydrate, high caloric, fatty foods, which raises serotonin, and makes that whole thing settle.

This is why the first thing I do with my clients is to find out what their sleeping situation is like, and immediately improve it. This is your key to optimal fat burning, perfect health, and longevity. The best part about sleep is that it's free.

Melatonin is a hormone (and antioxidant) which increases your body's ratio of this fat-burning fat (BAT). If you're not getting quality sleep, then you're putting yourself at a metabolic disadvantage, because you're not allowing your body to produce this powerful hormone and antioxidant.

There's a ton of research showing that many health conditions will get worse if you are not getting at least seven hours of quality sleep every night. You cannot have perfect health without quality sleep. Sleep is the foundation that perfect health is built on; without it, the house will fall apart, wall by wall.

Tools for Better Sleep

I'm about to unload an arsenal of effective tools for you to begin implementing, so that you can upgrade your sleep, tonight! You can pick and choose which tool you want to use, or you can use them all. The more tools you use, the better results you'll get.

Let's dig in.

Turn Your Bedroom into a Sleep Cave

Add these few changes to your bedroom for a significant increase in sleep.

Adjust the temperature. Studies have found that in general, the optimal temperature for sleep is quite cool, between 60 and 68 degrees Fahrenheit. Temperatures in this range help facilitate the decrease in core body temperature that in turn initiates sleepiness. Temperatures that fall too far below or above this range can lead to restlessness. A growing number of studies are finding that temperature regulation plays a role in many cases of chronic insomnia.

Researchers have shown, for example, that insomniacs tend to have a warmer core body temperature than normal sleepers just before bed, which leads to heightened arousal and a struggle to fall asleep.

Consider purchasing the ChiliPad™ Cube. This is a mattress pad with a cooling and heating temperature control system. It regulates the surface temperature of your mattress by actively circulating water through a network of microtubes. You can find it at chilitechnology.com.

Turn off electronics at least one hour before bed. This may be the hardest tip to follow. You read from your Kindle, check your email, text friends—all while trying to fall asleep. Many experts feel that our excessive use of communications technology (e.g., cell phones, laptops, television) is correlated with a significant increase in sleep deprivation. It's no wonder so many Americans struggle with poor sleep since 95 percent have reported using some type of electronics at least a few nights a week within the hour before bed.

Make your room as dark as possible. Unplug everything that glows and cover your windows with black curtains. Yes, it might feel like you are about to begin a 3-month hibernation, but you'll sleep like a baby.

Research has shown that nighttime light exposure suppresses the production of melatonin, which is the major hormone secreted by the pineal gland that controls sleep and wake cycles. Therefore, it would make sense that a reduction in melatonin at night is associated with subjective levels of sleeplessness. But melatonin suppression has far worse consequences than simply poor sleep outcomes: it has also been shown to increase the risk of cancer, impair immune system function, and possibly lead to cardio-metabolic consequences such as type 2 diabetes, metabolic syndrome, obesity, and heart disease. This is some serious business.

Listen, if you are not willing to shut down the MacBook, or power down the iPhone, at least reduce the brightness on the screen.

I want you to consider that you need a heart rate of 60 beats per minute or below to enter into a state of unconsciousness. Each time you reach for your phone and see a stimulating video or comment, it will elevate your heart rate, making it that much harder to fall asleep and stay asleep. Avoid engagement. Stay away from anything that arouses you. Set your cell phone on "airplane mode." Anything you can do to reduce electromagnetic frequencies (EMFs) is a great idea.

A great book all about EMFs is *The Non-Tinfoil Guide to EMFs: How to Fix Our Stupid Use of Technology,* by Nicolas Pineault.

Wean the bean: Have a caffeine curfew. If you are a regular reader of mine, you know how much I love my coffee—specifically, my fatty keto coffee as it puts my mind into an amazing place where I become more productive and perform better.

However, you need to let your mind rest after its high output performances. Due to the long half-life of caffeine—five to eight hours—even drinking coffee six hours or more before bedtime can have dramatic effects. In one study, participants consumed caffeine six hours before bedtime, and physiological measurements showed they lost on average an hour of sleep a night, even though the subjects weren't aware of it themselves.

As a rule of thumb, you should wean the bean after 2:00 p.m. I know some of you reading this are thinking, "Dude, I can have a shot of espresso and fall asleep just fine."

My reply would be, "That doesn't mean the sleep you are getting is quality, restorative sleep!"

Having a caffeine curfew will make sure you get all of the cognitive benefits of caffeine without sacrificing your sleep. Some people need more than eight hours of caffeine avoidance to sleep with maximum performance.

Take advantage of your "money time sleep window." There's a magical process called "money time sleep window." One hour of sleep within this window is equivalent to two hours of sleep outside of this window. It's all about recovery, repair, and rejuvenation.

This is based on our circadian rhythm. Our hormones are pretty damn predictable. We already established that the job of hormones is to communicate with other hormones, so they can complete the job of having your body function normally. This is exactly what perfect health is. When your body is functionally normal, you are creative, you have great energy levels, you can deal with any problem that comes your way, and it feels like you have superpowers.

Our hormones are in sync with Mother Nature. When the sun comes up, hormonal processes happen in the human body. When the sun goes down, other hormonal processes happen in the human body. As I mentioned, they are pretty damn predictable. Money time sleep window is based on a few hours after the sun has gone down, which is estimated to be 10:00 pm to 2:00 am. It varies depending on where you live in the world, but this is a great estimation.

The person seeking perfect health takes advantage of this window and prioritizes sleep during this period.

As Matthew Walker said, "Sleep is the single most effective thing we can do to reset our brain and body health each day— Mother Nature's best effort yet at contra-death."

Take a look at the super-successful entrepreneur Eric Thomas, aka The Hip Hop Preacher. This man grinds. He has been quoted saying "Sleep is for broke people! If you are willing to be successful, you have to be willing to give up sleep." Eric wakes up at 3:00 am every day. But here's the kicker: he goes to bed at 9:30 pm every night. Eric is harnessing the power of money time sleep window whether he knows it or not. You actually manufacture time! This is a slight edge hack that will take you to the next level.

Arnold Schwarzenegger said, "I've always figured out that there are 24 hours a day. You sleep for six hours and have 18 hours left. Now, I know there are some of you out there that say well, wait a minute, I sleep eight hours or nine hours. Well, then, just sleep faster, I would recommend."

How do you sleep faster? Money time sleep window.

"It is a common experience that a problem difficult at night is resolved in the morning after the committee of sleep has worked on it."– John Steinbeck

You snooze, you lose. Hitting the snooze button is the worst thing that's ever happened to sleep, according to America's Sleep Doctor, Michael Breus. The average snooze button is somewhere between 7-9 minutes in duration. Your body physically can't get into a deep stage of sleep during that short amount of time, so all that you are doing by hitting that snooze button each time is giving yourself crappy light sleep.

Do yourself a favor and stop using the snooze.

If you want to be the most productive person you know, you should never hit the snooze button. Here's a piece taken from the awesome book, *The 5 Second Rule* by Mel Robbins:

"There's actually a neurological reason why. I bet you didn't know that how you wake up is just as important as how you sleep. Scientists have recently discovered that when you hit the snooze button, it has a negative impact on brain function and productivity that can last up to four hours!

"We sleep in cycles that take about 90 to 110 minutes to complete. About two hours before you wake up, these sleep cycles end, and your body will start to slowly prepare to wake up. When your alarm goes off, your body is in wakeup mode. If you hit the snooze button and drift back to sleep, you force your brain to start a new sleep cycle that is 90 to 110 minutes long."

The problem, says Robbins, is that when the alarm rings again a few minutes after you've hit "snooze," the cortical region of your brain—the part responsible for decision-making, attention, alertness, and self-control—is still in the sleep cycle. It won't be able to snap awake, because it needs 75 more minutes to finish the sleep cycle you started.

As you drag yourself through the day, it can take up to four hours for this feeling of "sleep inertia" to wear off and for your cognitive functions to return to their full capacity. That's why when you get up after hitting the snooze, you feel like a bag of cement is in your head. It's not because you didn't get enough sleep. It's because once you hit the snooze button, you started a new sleep cycle and then interrupted it.

Try Mel Robbin's 5-Second Rule: After waking up, count down from 5, 4, 3, 2, 1, and then launch yourself out of bed. When you practice this technique consistently, you'll rewire your brain to teach your body to move every time you countdown to 1.

If you want to learn more about it, read her awesome book. Make it a non-negotiable rule: stop hitting the damn snooze button!

How to Become a Napping Ninja

Chronic fatigue is no joke. In America alone, millions of people suffer from debilitating tiredness and fatigue every single day. We resort to coffee, sugar, and stimulants just to get by, and feel awake enough to function. In this chapter, you'll discover tips to kick your afternoon energy slump, for good.

If you look at when you nap, what time of day, you can program what type of sleep you get. The perfect time of day to take a nap is between 1:00 pm and 3:00 pm in the afternoon. If you notice yourself getting sleepy or drowsy between these hours, this is because there's a slight core body temperature dip at that time, and that dip is very similar to the core body temperate drop that occurs around 10:30 pm at night, which is a signal to your brain to release melatonin (sleep hormone). This is why, in the afternoon, many people reach for that latte or 4-hour energy drink.

15 Essential BioHacks for Great Sleep

"Sleep is the chief nourisher in life's feast." — Matthew Walker

As an entrepreneur, I'm always looking for ways to increase my productivity. This is why biohacking is a favorite subject of mine. Two of my mentors are pros at biohacking: Dave Asprey and Ben Greenfield.

Biohacking (verb and noun) means:

(v): To change the environment outside of you and inside of you so you have full control of your biology, to allow you to upgrade your body, mind, and your life.

(n) The art and science of becoming superhuman.

This chapter is designed to help you achieve double the results, in half the amount of time. Here's a list of incredible life-transforming sleep biohacks. Enjoy, my fellow nerd!

BioHack #1: Leverage Your Natural Cortisol

Do not drink coffee again until you've read this!

You are about to discover the best time to have coffee. When you wake up in the morning, you get a natural surge in cortisol levels. Back in the day, when our ancestors encountered a lion or tiger, their bodies produced cortisol for a surge of energy to deal with the threat. Our ancestors had a decision to make: Fight this beast or run far away. In this day and age, we aren't encountering beasts in the wild, at least most of us aren't. So, the cortisol we produce provides us with energy to crush meetings, presentations, sports games, and performances. Cortisol is so powerful that caffeine pales in comparison to its potency. Since cortisol is elevated when you wake up, any caffeine taken within 90 minutes is pretty much rendered useless. Here's a cool hack: at about the 90-minute mark after rising, our cortisol begins to dip down. If you wait for that natural morning cortisol to dip down, and then you have your caffeine, it will actually help lift you into a higher energetic state. This is the golden time for coffee.

BioHack #2: Sun Lamp "Alarm Clock"

So many of us are jolted out of bed by an annoying alarm clock via our smartphone. When wear hear this dreaded alarm clock, we lift ourselves out of bed and are on automatic pilot. Over the years, I made the switch to a sun simulation lamp. This has been a gamechanger for me. If I want to be up at 7:00 am, the lamp will slowly light itself up around 6:30, getting a bit brighter by the minute. This simulates the natural way of waking up with the sun. It's a powerful way to control your morning, and not have your alarm control you. I personally use this lamp by Philips.

Hydrate after waking up. You breathe out through humidity about a liter of water each night during sleep. Let me rephrase that: you lose about one liter of water each night! Every living cell in your body needs water to function properly. Dehydration results in brain fog, muscle fatigue, and an entire host of symptoms. The very first thing you should do is drink 16 ounces of water as soon as you wake up. Add a pinch of high-quality salt to replenish your electrolytes. My favorite salt is Redmond's Real Salt.

BioHack #3: If You Think It, Ink It

Have you ever had the best ideas in the middle of the night? There're pens that have lights on them so you can click it and jot down that idea. Incredible.

BioHack #4: Stick to the Same Bedtime and Wake-up Time

Wake up time is more important. This means if you wake up at 6:30 am during the weekdays, you should wake up at the same time over the weekend. The more consistent you are with your circadian rhythm, the better off you are going to be.

BioHack #5: Mouth Taping for Deep Phases of Sleep

I know this sounds a little "woo woo," but I'm telling you there's science to back this up. Sealing your lips shut with tape while you sleep comes with a host of health benefits, including better sleep.

Strapping tape over your trap before bed encourages nasal breathing.

Studies reveal that nasal breathing is far superior to mouth breathing. It promotes better focus, memory, and concentration. Meanwhile, mouth breathing causes high blood pressure, heart problems, and sleep apnea.

Nasal breathing increases nitric oxide production in the sinuses, which is linked to healthy blood pressure levels, reduced inflammation, improved sleep, greater gains in endurance and strength, better memory, and even improved immune function.

Simply put: If you breathe through your mouth, you miss all of the benefits of the nitric oxide in your nose.

Check out the mouth-sealing sleep strips by Somnifix.

BioHack #6: Take a Cool, Not Cold, Shower After Waking Up

Have the shower head hit you square in the face, and focus on breathing. Leave for about a minute as it shunts all of the blood to your torso, which is very alerting. Total clarity after you get out of the shower!

BioHack #7: Upgrade Your Lighting

For the day: Install the Good Day Light Bulb by Lighting Science inside your bathroom, office, etc. Using the Good Day Light during the morning and afternoon hours can help your body naturally become more awake and alert. The Good Day Light Bulb provides an enriched blue light spectrum that mimics natural sunlight. When our bodies are exposed to blue light, the metabolic process to create melatonin (the sleep hormone) is stopped, and we feel naturally energized.

For the night: Install the Good Night Light Bulb by Lighting Science. The good night LED light bulb, originally developed for NASA astronauts on the international space station, lets melatonin do its thing and helps to regulate your body's natural circadian rhythm. So, when you're ready to sleep, your body is too.

BioHack #8: Once Every Year, Purchase a New Bed and Pillows

If you're sleeping on a worn-out pillow, scrunching and folding it up every night to get comfortable, that's a red flag that it's time to update. Even if your pillow isn't old and deflated, it might not be the best choice for your comfort and support. Dr. Michael Breus always says a good sleeping posture is key to sleeping soundly, night after night, and to waking without pain and stiffness. Your pillow helps to support a healthy sleep posture. If your neck and shoulders don't get sufficient support or are propped at an angle that causes twisting, craning, or crunching, this puts your spine and body out of alignment, leading to strain and discomfort in your neck, shoulders, and back, as well as sleeplessness.

When you consider that you spend 7 to 9 hours per night sleeping, that's over 2,500 hours per year that you spend in bed. Your physical, mental, and emotional performance are all directly correlated to the quality of the time spent on that bed, and a big part of that quality is the surface you're sleeping on: *your mattress.*

My favorite sleep mattress is from Samina Sleep, check them out here: www.saminasleep.com/ketokamp.

BioHack #9: Birth Control for Your Head

I'm talking about blue blocker glasses. If you want to be mentally sharp and be able to get deep sleep, then get yourself a pair of blue blocker glasses to wear. My girlfriend Natassia makes fun of me when I wear them at night—she calls them birth control for my head, but it's totally worth it.

When the sun goes down, we are designed to prepare for sleep. With so much stimulation around us at night in the form of blue light, we have literally manufactured a new daytime; this surprises melatonin and increases cortisol. This is the exact opposite of the hormonal process we want at night. With blue blockers and the Good Night Light Bulbs, you can prevent this unwanted process from happening. This allows your body to get ready for deep restorative sleep, which helps your brain filter our unwanted data from the day. When you do this consistently, it feels like you have superpowers because you become mentally clear, and a creative genius.

The brands I recommend are Swanwick Sleep and TrueDark.

A great book on brain health, sleep, and light exposure is *Headstrong,* by Dave Asprey.

BioHack #10: Yes—Keep the TV On!

If having your television on helps you fall asleep, then it's okay to leave your television on at night. But be sure to set a timer for it to shut off shortly after you fall asleep, otherwise it will wake you up during your normal cycle of light sleep. Also, make sure the television isn't too close to your bed; give yourself about six feet if possible.

BioHack #11: If Your Partner Snores, Mute 'Em!

Overcoming the torture of a snoring partner can be challenging! There's a superb product called Mute, which is a soft plastic internal nasal dilator designed to reduce snoring by gently opening nasal passages and preventing airway collapse. It's cheap, and it may even save your marriage.

Do you live in an area where sound keeps you up at night, or is your partner unwilling to use the Mute product? Then I have the perfect solution for you.

BioHack #12: Earplugs

Earplugs come in many designs and materials. It's important to determine whether you wish the earplug to fit into the ear canal or to cover your ear. Both techniques can block out sound.

What works best for you will probably be determined by fit. Ill-fitting earplugs won't provide you with enough noise reduction.

The size of your ear canal is an important factor. If the earplugs are too big for your ear canal, then they'll constantly slide out. Experimenting with different types may help you find the type that provides you with the most comfort and noise reduction.

Make sure to get the foam noise level rated at 32 or below because it drowns out about 30 decibels and you can still hear the smoke alarm if it goes off.

BioHack #13: Banana Tea Is Nature's Nyquil

Have you heard of banana tea before? I heard about it from Dr. Michael Breus. It turns out, the peel of the banana has more potassium and magnesium than the banana itself.

Here's how you make it:

Grab an entire organic banana. Leave the peel on, cut the ends off. Place it in a pot with 3-4 cups water. Boil until the peel turns brown, and then pour the water into a cup. This is keto friendly.

BioHack #14: Track Your Biometrics

Don't guess, test! The ultimate device for tracking your sleep, and much more, is the Oura Ring, at ouraring.com. It tracks key biometric data from your body, delivering critical insights to help you build good habits and harness your body's potential every day.

BioHack #15: My Top Five Sleep Supplements

Supplements are not created equal. There is a vast difference between synthetic supplements and the whole-food sourced variety.

When you take synthetic vitamins, the human body recognizes this substance as a drug. What results is expensive urine. When you take real food supplements, the human body recognizes this as nutrition. What results is something called selective absorption; this is when the body fills in any nutritional gaps, and excretes the rest.

My top five are magnesium glycinate, reishi mushroom, CBD oil, Gaba, and Sandman.

Visit ketokampkit.com to see my favorite sleep supplements and devices.

Zepiour's Story

For many years, Zepiour had been dealing with polycystic ovary syndrome (PCOS), hormone issues, and weight loss resistance. She came to me confused about nutrition and intermittent fasting. When we first met, it had been over a year since she had her period. Zepiour had numerous issues that interfered with her body's capability to heal. She enrolled into my Keto Kamp Academy, where she learned many of the tools from this book. After 28 days, I was scrolling through our private online group forum, and Zepiour shared an incredible victory. She shared that after 28 days of following the Keto Kamp plan, her monthly period came back. Her energy levels increased, her inflammation decreased, and—as a bonus side effect—she dropped 20 pounds of fat.

Hers is just one of many inspiring examples of the body's incredible ability to heal itself once you remove the toxic interference.

Chapter 12: Keto and Fasting for Women

What you've learn so far is that there is no cookie cutter approach to keto and fasting. You are unique, like a snowflake.

I want to share quick story to emphasize this. Every week, a teenage boy would walk by and see an artist going to work chipping away at a piece of stone. Several weeks into this, the artist had carved out a Greek god, a beautiful masterpiece of art. The teenage boy was astonished by what this artist was able to accomplish. The boy walked up to the artist and said, "Mister, how did you know this person was in there?"

The artist looked at him smiled and said, "Young man, he was in there the entire time."

Every human being has unique biochemical individual needs. Why is the Mona Lisa so expensive? This is because the Mona Lisa is one of a kind. It is unique in this world.

You are unique! You are one of a kind. You are a masterpiece because you are a piece of the master.

As a woman, you have a different number of hormones than men. When applying these ancient healing strategies there's special considerations for you. This is why I decided to dedicate an entire chapter for you.

Once you complete the Third Pillar, then you can start on the strategies in this chapter. It will provide you with a complete guide for how to use keto and fasting whether you are a cycling woman, peri-menopausal, or post-menopausal. I want to give credit where it's due for this research I'm about to share with you. Dr. Mindy Pelz, Dr. Stephanie Estima, Dr. Caitlin Czezowski, Dr. Sonya Jensen, Cynthia Thurlow and Dr. Daniel Pompa have really helped me understand how to apply keto and fasting to women.

Let's start with the ladies who currently have a monthly cycle.

What does your period say about your health?

Dr. Stephanie Estima said on The Keto Kamp Podcast, "Your monthly bleed is your hormonal report card." Your menstrual cycle is going to tell you about your hormonal status inside your body. If you have very heavy bleeding, heavy clotting, mood swings, bloating, or sleep disturbances, this is your body's way of telling you to pay attention. This is your body communicating to you. Symptoms are not the problem; it is feedback from your amazing body.

For women who are in their reproductive years, it's important to think about this hormonal milieu throughout the month. For simplicity's sake, we are going to break this up into 7-day cycles.

The first thing to do is track your monthly cycle. There are several apps you can use to track your monthly cycle. Clue is a good one (go to helloclue.com).

When you look at the first 7 days after the monthly cycle, the bleed week, the hormonal landscape is as follows. Most hormones are taking a break. Estrogen is low, testosterone is low, luteinizing hormone and progesterone are low. The one hormone that is elevated is follicular stimulating hormone (FSH), and its job is to continue to develop the follicle to help the one lucky egg to be released this month. During this follicular phase (7 days), you are more resilient to macro nutrient restriction. I suggest you follow a macronutrient approach of 70 percent fat, 25 percent protein, 5 percent carbohydrates. This is the optimal time to do a one-meal-a-day approach or even an extended block fast (3+ days). Since progesterone is not around during this week, your appetite won't be stimulated. This makes is much easier to do keto and fasting.

The second week, which is the week before ovulation, is leading up to the main event of releasing the egg whether you want to have a child or not. During this week we see a couple of hormones make their debut, estrogen becomes a rising star here. The concentration of estrogen increases significantly from week 1 to week 2. Estrogen is anabolic which helps with growth. The body increases estrogen here with its main to do develop the follicle so that you can release the egg.

The other hormone that makes a star debut here is testosterone. Your interest in sex and libido increases here. This makes sense because if you are having sex ahead of your ovulation the chances increase of a sperm meeting the egg. The number one priority for the body is survival and reproduction. If your body prioritizes cortisol, it won't make progesterone efficiently. All fasts have a cortisol response via a hormetic stress. This can be great during the first 14 days after the cycle, but not so good the 7 days leading up to the period. More yoga, walks, and slowing down with your workouts during the 7 days leading up to your period.

This time (day 6-13) is the best time to strength train. Building bone density and lean muscle mass is key for longevity in women. Resistance training would be terrific here in combination with protein. Protein stimulates mechanistic target of rapamycin (mTOR), which is the opposite of autophagy, which you have learned is catabolic, as it breaks down and recycles damaged cell components. This is why I recommend you change your macros to the following:

About 40 percent should come from fat, 45 percent should come from protein, and a slight increase in carbohydrates up to 15 percent. Your fasting schedule would shift to an 18/6 schedule with 2 meals within your 6-hour eating window.

This brings up to week 3. This is after ovulation. The entire hormonal landscape changes once again. I suggest you return to the week 1 guidelines. Your macronutrient approach of 70 percent fat, 25 percent protein, 5 percent carbohydrates. Now is when you want to be less restrictive with keto and fasting. Your fasting schedule changes to a 14/10 schedule with 3 meals during your 10-hour eating window.

The magic of resistant starches. During weeks 3 and 4, we see progesterone rise, which helps stimulate appetite and slow down your bowel movement. A resistant starch is a starch that resists digestion. The microbiota in the small intestine does not break them down. These starches enter the large intestine and become a food source for the microbiota in the large intestine. When you provide the large intestine with this fuel, it provides you a gift called butyrate, a short chain fatty acid. This helps with your sleep and cravings, and helps to repair the lining of the gut. The wonderful thing about the resistant starches is that they don't technically count toward your carbohydrate intake—they are essentially "free" carbohydrates. Woohoo!

As the Bulletproof Diet noted, there are four types of resistant starches:

RS1: Embedded in the coating of seeds, nuts, grains, and legumes.

RS2: Resistant granules in green bananas and raw potatoes.

RS3: This type transforms into resistant starch when cooked and then cooled, such as white potatoes and white rice.

RS4: Man-made resistant starch, such as contained in a manufactured, processed food like bread or cake. The label might say "polydextrin" or "modified starch." Synthetic isn't always a bad thing—one study found that a soluble fiber called resistant dextrin improved insulin resistance in women with type 2 diabetes.

Here are Keto Flex approved resistant starches:

• Green bananas

• Green banana flour

• Green plantains

• Green plantain flours

• Raw potatoes

• Raw potatoes starch

• Cold rice

The benefits of resistant starches include:

Reduces insulin resistance. Since resistant starch isn't digested, your insulin doesn't rise like other starches and cause blood sugar problems.

Protects against colon cancer. In a research study using mice, resistant starch killed precancerous cells in the gut and shrank cancerous lesions in the bowel.

Improves sleep. Resistant starch can also help you get better sleep. A 2017 study found that rats fed prebiotics had better non-REM sleep (the restorative phase) than rats who weren't given prebiotics.

Burns fat and curbs hunger. Resistant starch could help you control your weight. One study found that adding resistant starch to meals could make you feel fuller quicker, causing you to eat fewer calories. Another found that women who ate pancakes made with a resistant starch plus protein burned more fat after the meal than women who ate pancakes without resistant starch.[36]

Now we move into the fourth week. This is show time! Progesterone reaches its peak on day 21 and day 22. If you did blood work during this week, you'll see most things are down. You would see the following things reduced: blood glucose, amino acids, glutathione, lipids, and vitamin D. This is because your body is literally taking all of your substrates for energy and throwing it into your endometrium to thicken the lining and get you ready.

---

[36] Bulletproof.com. https://www.bulletproof.com/diet/bulletproof-diet/resistant-starch/

This is the best week to flex out of ketosis and increase your caloric load.

I recommend the following macronutrient changes: 50 percent of your total calories should come from healthy carbohydrates, 25 percent protein, 25 percent fat. Total calories should also increase by 10-15 percent. If you don't do this, you are going against your physiology, and Mother Nature always gets the last laugh, as you might find yourself elbow-deep in a bag of chips or ice cream bin.

My favorite carbohydrates for you at this time are squash, sweet potatoes, yams, yucca, citrus fruits, and ancient grains. You can find an entire list at the end of this book.

Perimenopause, Menopause & Post-Menopause

To the menopausal women: You are beautiful. You are not forgotten. Your wisdom and wrinkles are badges of honor. Let's discuss how keto and fasting applies to you.

When you are post-menopausal you can transfer all of the energy that would be used building up the uterine lining every month for something else. These are your golden years, ladies!

As you move from later stages of peri-menopausal to post-menopausal you tend to become more insulin resistant. What this means is that your cells are not as sensitive to the effect of insulin; insulin will have a harder time doing its job. Muscles also become resistant through anabolic resistance, which means it takes more for muscle to grow. This is where we see testosterone, estrogen, and other hormones drop down, which can result in symptoms. This means you have to work harder to maintain what you have.

When you are over 40, you literally have an organ that is shutting down—the ovaries. There's no other time in your life that this happens unless you have an organ removed. The ovaries make estrogen, progesterone and testosterone. This job is handed off the of adrenal glands.

A keto approach is wonderful here with the caveat of cyclical protein. Here's how you would do it. Here is a 28-day protocol for the perimenopausal, menopausal and post-menopausal woman:

Week 1: Keto macros 80 percent fat, 15 percent protein, 5 percent carbohydrates with an 18/6 intermittent fasting schedule.

Week 2: Keto macros 65 percent fat, 30 percent protein, 5 percent carbohydrates with an 18/6 intermittent fasting schedule. This is a great week to pair with strength training. This will help with the osteoblastic (bone growth) and osteoclastic (breaking down) ratio to maintain muscle mass and bone density for longevity. My favorite exercises are squats, push-ups, shoulder press, walks with your dog. My friend Giancarlo Anzellotti has a great YouTube channel with workout videos at youtube.com/gc3fitness.

Week 3: Keto macros 80 percent fat, 15 percent protein, 5 percent carbohydrates with an 18/6 intermittent fasting schedule.

Week 4: The 5-1-1 rule. This is a great week to pair with strength training.

• 5 days of intermittent fasting for 16 to 20 hours. When you are eating during the 4- to 8-hour window, stick to a ketogenic (high healthy fats) approach. Keto macros 80 percent fat, 15 percent protein, 5 percent carbohydrates.

• 1 day, complete a 24-hour water-only fast (dinner to dinner).

• 1 day, complete a feast day. Have three meals of high (healthy) carbohydrates and/or protein. Consume at least 150 grams of healthy carbs and/or protein. Eat less fat on this day.

Another thing to consider is that estrogen tends to decrease during menopause, and while you may no longer have this estrogen production from the ovaries, you can improve this through resistance training. Stress is an important component here, because after menopause your main source of estrogen will be from your adrenal glands.

Laura's Story

"I did not expect that I could ever have emotional freedom in my food and eating, because I had been so regimented," said Laura in her video testimonial about her experience at Keto Kamp. At age

59, Laura considered herself to be a "professional dieter," who from the age of 13 had been on one diet or another. She recognized she had an eating disorder, which she felt was controlling her life. As a beauty queen with a shelf full of trophies, Laura knew she was dieting "not for health, but for looks." There's a difference! When the beauty business faded and menopause hit her at age 54, she changed her focus to eating for health. She wrote down on paper, "My goal is extreme health." She wanted to be healthy not only for herself but for her three daughters. But she was misguided; she ate many small meals throughout the day, and these meals included lots of carbohydrates. Guess what? She felt hungry all the time, and especially at night. (This problem is very common!) She realized she was burning sugar, and it was better to burn fat. She went online and found a video of a guy with "Keto Kamp" on the wall behind him. (That would be yours truly.) She was intrigued. She gave my keto diet a half-hearted try by cutting sugar and eating more fat, but that didn't work. As she told me, "I realized this isn't about how I *eat*, but how I *live*." She began to work on every aspect of her health, including her sleeping and her mind-body connection, and today, she's never felt better. She likes my Keto Kamp Academy program because she's found that we "put it all together," like a one-stop shop that has all the resources you need to live a longer, healthier life.

Chapter 13: Apply What You've Learned

Having gotten this far in the book, you might find yourself feeling overwhelmed with the information I've presented, almost like you've been blasted by a firehose of ideas.

Not to worry—this chapter provides easy steps for you to apply the principles you've learned.

Look at your health as like a bucket. When you're born into this world, your bucket is mostly empty. It's very lightweight and easy to carry. As you continue through life, your bucket gets filled up with a poor diet, negative thoughts ("stinkin' thinkin'"), toxins, and other lifestyle factors. As your bucket gets fuller and heavier, you start to experience symptoms. You may not have thought of them this way, but symptoms are gifts from the body. They signal to you that something is awry, and that action is needed. In your car, you wouldn't ignore your check engine light, right? The truth is that many people do ignore their symptoms, or they mask them with pills, supplements, or even elective surgery.

If your bucket continues to get full, eventually it overflows, leading to a serious problem.

This book is intended to teach you how to empty out your bucket by focusing on the underlying causes of your symptoms.

Take it one step at a time. If you need to, go back and review the chapters. Which solution did you feel like you could tackle first? If you can say, "Hey, I can do that!" then go ahead and try.

I wrote this book to empower you to become a genius at managing your good health. The four pillars in Keto Flex will move you from a path of building disease to a path of building vitality.

If the self-guided, stepped approach doesn't work for you, I offer resources to make your journey much easier. I've built the Keto Kamp Academy, a friendly, supportive online community of people who are all working these principles. It's a fun and low-cost membership group where I teach keto and fasting variations. I've taken what you've learned in this book and put it together in a step-by-step system with video guidance. You also receive two monthly coaching calls with me.

Steps to Putting It All Together

1. Pick the lifestyle change you need the most.

2. Work the steps of that lifestyle change in the order I gave them through the four pillars.

3. Once you've mastered one pillar and lifestyle, move to the next lifestyle and pillar you are drawn to.

4. Work the pillars.

5. If you need more structure or community support, join the Keto Kamp Academy.

6. Get further tests or a health consultation to customize your needs.

If you still feel lost, please reach out to me. We have an amazing team here at Keto Kamp of caring people who are here to support you and get you in the right direction. Setbacks are inevitable, but it isn't about the setback, it is about the get back! You might need to do more testing to understand your body better. Wherever you are on your journey, just keep going. Too many people think it's impossible to heal based on their history and/or age, but this is a false belief. I want you to experience perfect health, and you will. Whether you work the steps in each pillar or join my keto Kamp Academy, know that I am rooting for you. Keto Flex is a scientifically proven way to rid your symptoms for good. When you understand how to correct your symptoms with changes made to your lifestyle, your body will heal. Let's take control over your health once and for all.

David's Story

David is 50 years old, and he says, "I feel amazing!"

It wasn't always that way. In fact, David spent most of his adult years feeling absolutely miserable.

Since the age of 17, he suffered from type 1 diabetes. As an adult, before he started his Keto Kamp Academy journey, David was in very poor health. He weighed 294 pounds and had a body mass index (BMI) of 42. (A BMI of 30 or greater is considered obese.) He was on 15 medications for depression, anxiety, and high blood pressure. His blood pressure was as high as 200/101, which is serious hypertension.

Other symptoms of poor health included rapid heartbeat (110 resting) and excessive sweating (he felt hot all the time). His blood sugar levels showed an A1C of 8.3, an indicator of significant diabetes. He used over 200 units of Novolog insulin every day, and had large spikes in his blood glucose levels.

He was in sad shape—no energy, low testosterone, taking ADD meds, suffering from acid reflux, and feeling very week. Each day seemed worse than the one before.

No one should have to live like that.

After following the steps outlined in the Keto Kamp Academy, David feels like he has a new lease on life. He now weighs 186 pounds and has a BMI of 26.7 percent—overweight, yes, but far better than being obese! Even better, he's off *all* those meds except 18-24 units of insulin a day.

His depression gone and his blood pressure is down to a normal reading of 112/72. His resting heart rate is down to 74, the excessive sweating is gone—he's even comfortable in summer heat —and he has an A1C of 4.7 with no blood glucose spikes. He has no more acid reflux.

David told me, "I have lots of energy. I'm never sick except seasonal allergies, and I feel amazing every day! I've intentionally come out of ketosis just times—the 4th of July, my November birthday, and Father's Day."

Here's David's chart:

He lost 94 pounds in 8 months. Macros: 75/20/5. Ketones: 2.5 - 6.0.

Then he had a complete stall at 200 pounds. Macros: 65/30/5. Ketones 0.3 - 2.0.

As of this writing, he had lost 14 pounds in the previous 3 months. Macros: 75/20/5. Ketones: 0.5 - 4.4.

He'd like to be 170 pounds with a BMI of 25 percent or less. I know he can do it!

Chapter 14: Shopping Lists, Fat Burning Keto Recipes & The Keto Kamp Blueprint

Here are some menus you can try at home, as well as a shopping list of keto-friendly foods for your refrigerator.

Breakfast

Low Carb Egg Salad

Ingredients:
- Twelve large, pastured eggs
- Half cup of Primal Kitchen Mayonnaise
- Two tablespoons of melted grass-fed butter
- One teaspoon of French's yellow mustard
- 1/3 cup of finely minced white onion
- One teaspoon of black pepper
- One teaspoon sea salt

Directions:
1. Fill a big pot with cold water, and place in the eggs. Heat the water until it boils, for 10 minutes.
2. Expel pot from heat and drain out as much of the hot water as you can. Leave the eggs in pot and refill it with cool water.
3. Allow the eggs to sit in cold water for two to three minutes.
4. Take out the eggs, pat them dry, and peel them.
5. Chop the peeled eggs into uniform quarter inch pieces. You can also make use of an egg slicer.

6. Include the rest of the ingredients and combine thoroughly. Freeze until ready to eat.

Broccoli & Cheddar Egg Puffs

Ingredients:
- Eight pastured eggs at room temperature
- Two tablespoons grass-fed butter gently melted
- A quarter of cup heavy cream raw
- One teaspoon of Dijon mustard
- One tablespoon of nutritional yeast
- Half teaspoon of garlic powder
- Half cup of broccoli florets fresh, frozen, or leftover, chopped
- A quarter cup of Parmesan cheese, shredded
- A quarter teaspoon of sea salt
- Half cup of cheddar cheese shredded
- Add-ins like, mushrooms, asparagus, sausage, leftover chopped cooked meats bacon,
- peppers, kale, spinach, fresh herbs, etc.

Directions:
1. Preheat the oven to 350 degrees F.
2. If using a muffin pan, grease thoroughly. Or set out silicone muffin liners.
3. Whisk the eggs in a mixing bowl.
4. Add the melted grass-fed butter and whisk properly.
5. Add heavy cream. Whisk well.
6. Add nutritional yeast, sea salt, garlic powder, and Dijon mustard. Whisk thoroughly.
7. Add cheese and broccoli (or other add-ins). Sr to mix.
8. Fill muffin cups or liners 3/4 full.
9. Bake for about 25 to 30 minutes, or until the point when set and tops are lightly browned.
10. Enjoy!

Keto Pancakes

Ingredients:
- Four organic, pastured eggs
- Half teaspoon of pure vanilla extract
- Three tablespoons of coconut flour
- Four ounces of grass-fed cream cheese
- A quarter teaspoon of powdered stevia
- Pastured grass-fed butter or ghee

Directions:
1. Place all of your ingredients apart from the grass-fed butter / ghee into a blender, and blend until the mixture is smooth.
2. Pour the batter straight from the blender's pitcher into your frying pan which has been pre- heated and greased with grass fed butter.
3. As soon as bubbles appear uniformly across your low carb pancake, flip and cook until the other side is done.
4. Remove the pancake from the pan and move to a plate, then top with grass fed butter or ghee.

Keto Breakfast Burrito

Ingredients:
- Two tablespoons of unsweetened almond milk
- Ghee for greasing
- Four pastured eggs
- Four strips of cooked pasture-raised bacon, chopped
- One medium tomato, diced
- Fresh greens of your liking (spinach, cilantro, basil)
- Half avocado, sliced

Directions:
1. In a mixing bowl, whisk together the eggs and almond milk.
2. Heat a skillet over medium heat and daintily grease with ghee.
3. Pour half of the mixture into the pan to coat the base thinly. Seal and cook for 3 minutes. Use a spatula to move to a plate.

4. Pour the rest of the mixture into the skillet and cook for an extra 3 minutes, covered.

5. Top each egg "tortilla" with tomato, bacon, greens and avocado. Roll and enjoy!

Lunch

Keto Cobb Salad

Ingredients:
Salad
- Eight oz. of cooked Organic free-range chicken
- Four strips of uncured bacon
- Two free range eggs
- One Haas avocado
- Four cups of chopped Romaine lettuce
- Dressing
- One Haas avocado
- 1/3 cup of coconut milk
- One tablespoon of organic Dijon mustard
- Three tablespoons of extra virgin olive oil
- Two tablespoons of organic champagne vinegar
- Juice of one lemon
- One clove of garlic, pressed
- A quarter teaspoon of sea salt

Directions:
1. Put the eggs in a saucepan and cover with water. Heat to the point of boiling and simmer for 15 minutes. Deplete, chill, peel, and dice.
2. Meanwhile, cook the bacon over medium heat in a safe skillet. Put on the paper towels to drain, dice.
3. Dice the pre-cooked organic free-range chicken

4. Prepare the dressing. Put the avocado, olive oil, vinegar, mustard, coconut milk, lemon juice, garlic and sea salt in a blender. Blend thoroughly, adding water to achieve the desired consistency.
5. Chop the Romaine lettuce finely and divide among serving bowls.
6. Top with diced avocado, organic free-range chicken, egg and bacon. Drizzle with dressing.
7. Enjoy.

Avocado Chicken Salad

Ingredients:
- Two of cups poached Organic free-range chicken neatly diced (10 oz)
- One medium-sized Hass Avocado, mashed
- 1/3 cup of celery, finely diced
- Two tablespoons of red onion or scallion, minced
- Two tablespoons of cilantro, finely chopped
- Two tablespoons of extra virgin avocado oil
- One tablespoon of fresh lemon or lime juice
- Sea salt and pepper as seasoning

Directions:
1. Combine the celery, onion, and cilantro in a medium bowl. Dice the Organic free-range chicken and transfer to the bowl.
2. Chop through the avocado using a chef's knife until the blade hits the pit. Slide the knife around the pit, chopping the avocado into two equal parts. Twist the halves to divide them. Expel the pit by tapping the knife into the pit until it sticks. Ensure that the avocado half is held firmly on a cutting board before proceeding with it. Using a spoon, scoop out the avocado flesh and put into a little bowl. Mash until smooth and creamy using a fork. Stir in the lemon juice and oil.
3. Transfer the mashed avocado to the mixture and stir to combine. Enjoy on a low carb bagel or serve over lettuce.

Chili Lime Chicken

Ingredients:
- Three tablespoons of Extra Virgin Avocado Oil
- One tablespoon of Chili Powder
- Twelve Organic free-range chicken drumsticks
- One tablespoon of Garlic Powder
- One tablespoon of Lime Juice
- Sea salt as seasoning

Directions:
1. Combine the extra virgin avocado oil, chili powder, lime juice, and garlic powder in a large bowl until well mixed.
2. Transfer the Organic free-range chicken drumsticks into the mixture to uniformly coat.
3. Seal and allow to marinate for about 30-60 minutes.
4. Preheat the grill to a medium-high heat, while the organic free-range chicken is marinating.
5. Put the Organic free-range chicken on the grill grates and change sides at approximately 5 minutes intervals until the chicken temperature reaches 185F, about 30-40 minutes depending on size of drumsticks.
6. Add sea salt to taste.

Keto Baked Salmon with Avocado Salmon

Ingredients:
- Four wild caught salmon fillets
- One teaspoon of ground cumin
- One teaspoon of paprika
- Fresh cilantro, minced
- One teaspoon of onion powder
- Two teaspoon of chili powder
- Two tablespoon of lemon juice
- Two tablespoon of olive oil

- Sea salt and freshly ground black pepper
- Avocado Salsa Ingredients
- One tablespoon of fresh lime or lemon juice
- One avocado, peeled and diced
- Half cucumber, chopped
- Half bell pepper, diced
- Quarter cup of olive oil
- Half teaspoon of ground cumin
- Red onion, minced
- Sea salt and freshly ground black pepper

Directions:

1. Preheat the oven to 400 F.
2. Combine the cumin, paprika, onion powder and chili powder in a bowl; add sea salt and pepper as seasoning.
3. Brush the wild caught salmon fillets with the olive oil and lemon juice.
4. Sprinkle the wild caught salmon fillets with the spice mixture and put in a baking dish.
5. Bake for about 12 to 15 minutes in the oven.
6. Mix together all the ingredients for the avocado salsa in a small bowl.
7. Season the salsa with sea salt and pepper to taste, and gently mix until thoroughly mixed.

Keto Salmon Salad
Ingredients:

- Sea salt and black pepper as seasoning
- Half teaspoon of garlic powder
- One tablespoon of fresh lemon juice
- One six-ounce salmon fillets
- One tablespoon of olive oil
- Half cup of crumbled feta or blue cheese leave out for paleo or Whole 30
- Two avocados, peeled, pied, and chopped into slices

- Half cucumber sliced in rounds
- Four cups of chopped mixed green lettuce
- Two hard-boiled eggs, peeled and sliced
- Five slices of bacon, cooked and chopped
- One cup of grape or cherry tomatoes halved
- For the vinaigrette
- Three to four tablespoon of apple cider vinegar
- Two tablespoons of sour cream set aside for paleo
- One teaspoon of garlic powder
- Three tablespoons of extra virgin olive oil or extra virgin avocado oil
- Sea salt and pepper as seasoning

Directions:

1. Pat the salmon dry. Rub the two sides with extra virgin avocado oil and lemon juice. Season with sea salt, garlic powder, and pepper.

To Grill Salmon:

1. Preheat the grill to medium-high heat and cook for four-five minutes on the two sides or until the internal temperature is about 62 F. Using a fork, flake the cooked salmon into bite- sized pieces and put aside.

To Broil Salmon:

1. Heat the broiler and line a baking sheet with foil or parchment paper. Place the salmon on pan and broil for 8 to 10 minutes or till the point when the Wild Caught fish flakes easily when tested with a fork.

Prepare the salad:

1. Whisk all the ingredients for the vinaigrette together. Drizzle one teaspoon over the sliced avocado (to keep it from browning).
2. Add the lettuce in a large bowl, then top with flaked salmon, eggs, bacon, avocado, tomatoes, cucumber, and cheese. Drizzle with the dressing right before serving.

Ketogenic Avocado Fries

Ingredients:

For the fries

- Two large Haas avocados, peeled and pied
- Half teaspoon of sea salt
- Three tablespoons of extra virgin avocado oil for the dipping sauce
- A quarter cup of Primal Kitchen mayonnaise
- 3/4 teaspoon of sea salt
- A quarter teaspoon of apple cider vinegar for the garnish
- 1/8 teaspoon of dried parsley
- 1/8 teaspoon of ground black pepper

Directions:

1. Prepare the fries by chopping the avocados lengthwise— each avocado half should give you four or five strips. Spread the strips on a clean surface and sprinkle sea salt on it, concealing all sides.

2. Put the extra virgin avocado oil in a big frying pan and set the heat to medium. Heat for about 60 seconds.

3. Include the avocado strips to the hot oil and fry ll it turns golden on one side, around four minutes. Fry them in batches of two if desired so as not to overcrowd the pan. Flip each strip over carefully and repeat until all the strips are golden on every side. Move the finished fries to a clean plate and repeat with the rest of the uncooked fries.

4. Meanwhile, prepare the dipping sauce: mix together the Primal Kitchen mayonnaise with the sea salt and apple cider vinegar in a small bowl.

5. When all the fries are done, sprinkle with the pepper and parsley. Serve with the dipping sauce and enjoy!

Dinner

Keto Ground Beef Zucchini Boats
Ingredients:
- Two medium zucchinis (about 8 inches)
- 3/4 pound of 100% grass-fed ground beef
- One small onion, chopped
- Half cup of chopped fresh mushrooms
- Half cup of chopped sweet red pepper
- Half cup of chopped green pepper
- Half cup of shredded cheddar cheese, divided
- Two tablespoons of ketchup
- Sea salt and pepper as seasoning

Directions:
1. Trim the ends off the zucchini. Chop the zucchini in two equal parts lengthwise; scoop out pulp, leaving half inch's shells. Neatly chop the pulp.

2. Cook the beef, zucchini pulp, onion, mushrooms and peppers in a skillet over medium heat until the meat is no longer pink; drain. Take down from the heat. Thoroughly combine half cup of cheese, ketchup, sea salt and pepper. Spoon into the zucchini shells. Transfer to a greased 13×9 inches baking dish. Sprinkle with the rest of the cheese.

3. Bake, opened at 350° for 25-30 minutes or until zucchini is tender.

4. When scooping out the pulp for Zucchini Boats, a teaspoon is the most appropriate size. Use your food processor or blender to finely chop the pulp immediately.

Low Carb Keto Chili

Ingredients:
- Two ribs of celery, chopped
- Two lbs. 85/15 100% grass fed ground beef

- One teaspoon of sea salt
- One teaspoon of ground chipotle chili powder
- One tablespoon of chili powder
- Half tablespoon of avocado oil
- Two teaspoon of garlic powder
- One tablespoon of cumin
- One teaspoon of black pepper
- One fifteen oz. can of no salt-added tomato sauce
- One 16.2 oz. container of bone broth

Directions:
1. Pour the avocado oil in a large pot and heat over medium heat. Include the chopped celery and cook until so, about 3-4 minutes. Transfer the celery to a separate bowl and put aside.
2. Lower heat to medium-low, include beef bone broth and tomato sauce to cooked beef, and simmer covered for 10 minutes, stirring sporadically.
3. Transfer the celery back to the pot and stir until well combined.
4. Garnish, serve, and enjoy!

Keto Ground Beef & Spinach Skillet

Ingredients:
- One king oyster mushroom, chopped
- Two tablespoons of raw almonds, chopped
- 150g 100% grass fed ground beef
- Half teaspoon of chili pepper flakes
- Two tablespoons of coconut oil or ghee
- A pinch of Himalayan sea salt
- A pinch of ground white pepper
- A quarter cup of pitted kalamata olives
- One tablespoon of capers
- One tablespoon of all-natural roasted almond butter
- 150g baby spinach leaves, roughly chopped

Directions:

1. Dissolve the coconut or ghee in a heavy cast iron skillet set over medium-high heat. When the fat is nice and hot, include the chopped mushroom and cook around two to three minutes until golden and have a pleasant or sweet smell.

2. Include the chopped almonds and keep cooking for around a minute, then throw in ground beef, sea salt, white pepper and chili pepper flakes and cook until the meat is totally browned and cooked through, about five to six minutes.

3. Include olives, capers and almond butter and stir until thoroughly mixed. Finally, hurl the chopped spinach in and stir until it's totally wilted and thoroughly distributed.

4. Move to a bowl and serve immediately.

5. Garnish with crispy lardons.

Quick Tandoori Salmon

Ingredients:
- Two Wild Salmon Fillets - medium size
- One teaspoon of Ginger + Garlic Paste
- Half cup of 100% grass fed Greek Yogurt
- Two teaspoons of Olive Oil
- Half Lemon Juice

Spices for Tandoori Masala
- 1/8 teaspoon of Turmeric Powder
- One teaspoon of Coriander Powder
- One teaspoon of Red Kashmiri Mirch Powder
- One teaspoon of Garam Masala - mix of cloves, pepper, cardamoms, cinnamon
- One teaspoon of Dry Fenugreek Leaves
- One teaspoon of Cumin Powder
- Sea salt as seasoning

Directions:
1. Combine the yogurt, ginger/garlic paste, lemon juice and all spices in a large bowl.

2. Add the wild caught Salmon and put aside for 10 minutes.

3. Preheat the oven to 400-degree F.

4. Line a baking tray with foil and spray cooking oil.

5. Put the marinated wild caught salmon on the tray and bake for 15 minutes in the oven.

6. Then increase the heat to a broil and cook for 3-4 minutes until it begins to char on the surface.

7. Be very observant as this can burn quickly.

8. Turn off the oven and expel the baking tray.

9. Move over the salmon to serving dishes and serve immediately with mint chutney and vegetables.

10. (You can serve this dish with any side of your liking).

Keto Condiments

Homemade Cesar Salad Dressing

Ingredients:
- One egg yolk
- One tablespoon of anchovy paste
- Two tablespoon of lemon juice
- Two cloves of garlic
- One tablespoon of oregano
- Two teaspoons of Dijon mustard
- One teaspoon of sea salt
- One teaspoon of black pepper
- Half cup of light extra virgin olive oil
- Half cup of parmesan

Directions:
1. Add all of the ingredients in a food processor apart from the olive oil. Pulse for 30 seconds until it is well combined. Add olive oil in a slow stream while pulsing through the small hole on the cover of food processors designed for adding liquids. This will thicken the salad dressing.

2. Keep at this until you have added every drop of oil to the food processor. At this point, your dressing should be prey thick.
3. Add the parmesan and blend for twenty more seconds and you're all set!

Olive Oil and Balsamic Vinegar Salad Dressing
Ingredients:
* 1/3 cup of vinegar (balsamic)
* Two cloves of garlic minced.
* One half teaspoon of black pepper
* One half teaspoon of sea salt
* One tablespoon of Dijon mustard
* 2/3 cup of extra virgin olive oil

Directions:
1. Add the balsamic vinegar to a jar with a lid.
2. Add the garlic, pepper, and sea salt.
3. Put lid on mason jar and shake to mix dressing.
4. Place Dijon in next and shake again to mix.
5. Lastly, add the olive oil.
6. Allow to sit for about an hour so flavors are well combined.

Avocado Oil Mayonnaise

Ingredients:
* A quarter teaspoon of sea salt
* A quarter teaspoon of Dijon mustard
* Two egg yolks
* One teaspoon of lemon juice
* One teaspoon of white wine vinegar
* One cup of extra virgin avocado oil

Directions:
1. Put the egg yolks, vinegar, sea salt, lemon juice, and mustard in a container, and using an immersion blender, blend until thoroughly mixed and slightly thick, around 30 seconds.

2. Slowly put in the extra virgin avocado oil a little at a me while blending with the immersion blender. You may need to move the blender up and down to mix in the oil. It should begin to thicken immediately. Continue going until you've mixed one cup of oil, and at that point, stir thoroughly with a spatula. It should be exceedingly thick.

3. Store in a container and put in the refrigerator until needed.

Best Ways to Cook Food

* Raw
* Lightly Heated Steamed
* Baked at 320°F or below
* Simmered
* Boiled
* Poached
* Lightly grilled (not charred)
* Sous Vide
* Slow Cooking
* Pressure cooking

Worst Ways to Cook Food

* Broiled
* Barbecued
* Burnt
* Blackened
* Charred
* Deep Fried
* Microwaved

Avoid the Following Dirty Keto Foods

* Only remove these for the first 28 days

- Corn Oil
- Soybean Oil
- Fried Foods
- Factory chicken fat
- Sunflower oil
- Grain Fed Beef
- Farmed Fish
- Safflower oil
- Fish Oil
- Canola oil
- Cottonseed Oil
- Margarine
- Legumes (including peanuts and chickpeas) *
- Corn
- Raisins
- Dried fruit
- Jam
- Jelly
- Soy Milk
- Diet Drinks & Soda
- Burned/Blackened Meat
- Spinach*
- Almonds*
- Potato Starch*
- Organic Grass Fed Sour Cream*
- Grass Fed Heavy Cream*
- Powdered Milk
- Factory Dairy
- Nightshades (tomatoes, potatoes, goji berries, peppers, eggplant) *
- Soy (Except organic fermented soy such as natto & tempeh) *
- Dairy replacer
- Condensed or Evaporated Milk
- Conventional Ice Cream
- Wheat
- Corn
- Millet
- Potato Starch
- Corn Starch
- Garbanzo Flour

Approved Oils & Fats

- Coconut oil
- Pastured Egg Yolks
- Grass Fed Animal Fat & Marrow
- Avocado oil
- Grass-Fed Butter
- Sunflower Lecithin
- Grass-Fed Ghee
- Cacao Butter
- Brain Octane Oil
- XCT Oil
- Dark Chocolate
- Palm Oil
- Palm Kernel
- Extra-Virgin Olive Oil
- Pastured Bacon Fat
- MCT oil

Approved Nuts, Seeds & Legumes

* Only remove these for the first 28 days

- Coconut
- Coconut flour
- Almonds*
- Cashews*
- Chestnuts

- Hazelnuts
- Macadamia
- Pili Nuts
- Pecans
- Walnuts
- Sunflower seeds
- Almond Flour*
- Cashew Flour*
- Pecan Flour
- Walnut Meal/Flour
- Nut Butters (Except Peanut)
- Sunflower Seed Butter
- Pine nuts

Approved Proteins

- Grass-Fed Beef & Lamb
- Pastured Eggs & Gelatin
- Colostrum
- Collagen Protein
- Beef Gelatin
- Marine Collagen
- Wild Anchovies
- Wild Haddock
- Wild Sardines
- Wild Sockeye salmon
- Wild Summer Flounder

- Wild Trout
- Grass-Fed Whey
- Pastured Pork
- Pastured Duck & Goose
- Hemp Protein
- Bone Broth
- Organic Free-Range Poultry

Approved Fruit & Carbohydrates for Keto Flex Days

- Avocado

- Blackberries

- Coconut

- Cranberries

- Lemon

- Lime

- Raspberries

- Blueberries

- Pineapple

- Strawberries

- Tangerine

- Grapefruit

- Pomegranate

- Apple

- Apricot

- Cherries

- Figs

- Kiwifruit

- Lychee

- Nectarine

- Orange

- Peach

- Pears

- Plums

- Bananas

- Dates

- Grapes

- Guava

- Mango

- Melons

- Papaya

- Passion Fruit

- Plantain

- Watermelon

- Asparagus

- Bok choy

- Broccoli

- Brussels Sprouts

- Cauliflower

- Celery

- Cucumber

- Fennel

- Olives

- Cooked Kale

- Cooked Collards Cabbage

- Lettuce

- Radishes

- Spinach

- Summer Squash

- Zucchini

Approved Fruit & Carbohydrates for Keto Flex Days (continued)

- Cilantro
- Pumpkin
- Butternut Squash
- Sweet potato
- Yam
- carrot
- White Rice
- Cassava
- Taro
- Tapioca Flour/Starch
- Green Onion
- Leeks
- Arrowroot
- Resistant Starch Powder
- Plantain Flour
- Black Rice
- Wild Rice
- Brown Rice
- Artichokes
- Zucchini
- Winter Squash
- Green Beans

Approved Dairy

- Colostrum
- Grass-fed ghee or Butter*
- Grass-fed Cream*
- Grass-fed Sheep's Yogurt
- Full-fat, Raw A2 Milk or Yogurt Non-Organic*
- Grass-fed Cow cheese*
- Raw Sheep/Goat Cheese

Approved Keto Sweeteners

- Erythritol
- Pure Stevia
- Monk Fruit
- Non-GMO dextrose

Keto Flex Day Sweeteners

- D-Ribose
- Glucose
- Raw Honey
- Maple syrup
- Coconut sugar

Non-Approved Sweeteners

- Xylitol
- Maltitol
- Sorbitol
- Acesulfame potassium accsulfame
- Mannitol
- Aspartame
- Sucralose
- Saccharine

Beverages

- Unsweetened Tea
- Zevia soda
- Organic Coffee

- E-lyte Water
- Thorne Electrolyte Powder
- High quality water
- Dry Farm Wines
- Almond Milk*
- Coconut Milk
- Cashew Milk*
- Hazelnut Milk
- Macadamia Nut Milk

Approved on The Go Keto Foods

- Canned Sardines
- Oysters
- Sockeye Salmon
- Mackerel
- Anchovies
- Raw Macadamia Nuts
- Roasted Nori Seaweed Crackers
- Hard Boiled or Deviled Eggs
- Raw Coconut Butter
- Guacamole with EPIC Pastured Pork Rinds or Bacon 'Chips'
- Avocados
- Homemade Fat Bombs
- Grass Fed Cheese/ Yogurt
- Sugar-Free Jerky
- High-Fat Smoothies & Puddings
- Homemade Unsweetened Popsicles
- Plant Based Pea Protein Powder
- Bulletproof & EPIC Bars
- Paleo Valley Beef Sticks

Optimal Blood Glucose & Ketone Ranges

- Blood Ketones: 0.8 – 2.8 mmol/L
- Fasted Blood Glucose: 72-92 mg/dL

Advanced Testing…

1 Hour Post Prandial:

- Blood Ketones (same range above)
- Blood Glucose: 120 mg/dL or below

2 Hours Post Prandial:

- Blood Ketones (same range above)
- Blood Glucose: 100 mg/dL or below

Thank You!

I acknowledge you for completing this book. You now understand how your body works at the cellular level. At this point you've already seen your health transform. You've noticed increased energy and fat loss, better sleep and mental clarity, and many (if not all) of your symptoms are gone. Revisit this book as many times as you'd like. Mix and match the four pillars according to your liking.

If you'd like to receive health coaching from me, and become a part of an incredible online community, I recommend you become a Keto Kamp Academy member today.

Keto Kamp Academy members receive access to an online portal with over 200 videos in a complete step by step system. In addition, you'll receive two monthly health coaching calls from me. Accountability is the glue that ties your goals to your results. You can gain instant access to The Keto Kamp Academy today by heading to www.ketokampacademy.com.

I encourage you to share this book with a friend, family member and/or co-worker. Please leave the book a rating/review on Amazon.

I would love to connect with you online via my social media platforms.

Website: www.benazadi.com

Instagram: www.instagram.com/thebenazadi

Facebook: www.facebook.com/thebenazadi

YouTube: www.youtube.com/ketokamp

Twitter: www.twitter.com/thebenazadi

TikTok: @thebenazadi

Clubhouse: @thebenazadi

LinkedIn: www.linkedin.com/in/benazadi

Podcast: The Keto Kamp Podcast is available on all platforms worldwide.

Take a photo of you holding this book and use the hashtag **#KetoFlex** so I can see it and share it with my community. Until next time.

- Ben Azadi, Founder of Keto Kamp